STEP™ Foundation

Module 1

F1: First STEP™

Series editor: Professor Mike Larvin

The Royal College *of* Surgeons *of* England

Published by The Royal College of Surgeons of England

Registered Charity No. 212808

35–43 Lincoln's Inn Fields
London WC2A 3PE
http://www.rcseng.ac.uk

STEP™ Foundation ISBN, 1-904096-05-0

Module 1: F1 – First STEP™ ISBN, 1-904096-06-9

Designed by ChatlandSayer, London, UK

Typeset by The Royal College of Surgeons of England, London, UK

Printed by Latimer Trend and Company, Estover Road, Plymouth PL6 7PY, UK

Contents

Message from the College President

Welcome to the College's distance learning programme— *STEP™ Foundation*. This edition is a new venture designed to support all Foundation year trainees. STEP™ is a well established programme which has proved highly popular with trainees, and which has been updated and expanded regularly since 1994. The new landscape for postgraduate medical training presents many challenges to The Royal College of Surgeons of England, but one of our earliest responses was to extend learning and pastoral support to Foundation doctors rather than just those already embarked on a career in surgery.

The *STEP™ Foundation* edition has been designed to provide you with the knowledge base you will need to support the practical workplace-based training you will receive during your Foundation programme. It also addresses all of the practical competences required from the Foundation curriculum. If you do aspire to a career in surgery, mastering the goals contained within STEP™ Foundation will be a major stepping stone towards specialist surgical training.

As a Foundation trainee you are in a daunting stage of your career development, experiencing a wide range of novel clinical practice and new situations, and beginning to develop your ability to make your own professional judgements. The coherently structured knowledge base that STEP™ provides will build on your earlier education and training, but is relevant to your day to day work. It will help you to get the best from your Foundation programme, and to complete your assessments with confidence and success.

The Royal College of Surgeons of England is an internationally recognized centre for education, training, assessment and research. The Raven Department of Education has an unsurpassed reputation for the design and delivery of innovative knowledge and skills-based courses. Surgeons who are experts across a range of surgical and other specialties, together with dedicated educational advisers, have combined forces to develop *STEP™ Foundation*, blending the traditional printed material you are holding in your hands, with extensive complementary multimedia resources as well as learning and pastoral support. The *e*STEP™ Foundation website provides real-life case-based learning scenarios and online discussion; allows you to assess your progress at every stage (aligned to the new intercollegiate MRCS assessments); provides extended material and updates for STEP™ printed content; and basic science support. Support is provided online by 'working' surgical trainers and also by your peers. You will be kept updated on STEP™ Foundation and other College events, and most importantly, the far reaching changes in specialist surgical training as they evolve over the coming months.

This College aims to put the interests of patients at the heart of everything we do, and I firmly believe that the STEP™ Foundation edition supports that aim by providing you with the best possible basis at the very start of your career. I wish you well in your studies, and hope to see you at one of the STEP™ College Days.

Bernard Ribeiro, President, The Royal College of Surgeons of England

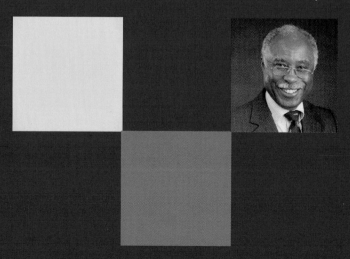

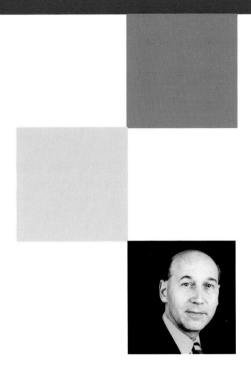

Message from the Series Editor

Welcome to this brand new *STEP^{TM} Foundation* edition of The Royal College of Surgeons of England's distance learning programme. STEP^{TM} – the Surgical Training and Education Programme – has been in existence since 1994, with a second edition in 1996 and a third in 2000. Each new edition was produced in response to changes in education and surgical training. The pace of these changes has quickened recently with the advent of the Modernising Medical Careers (MMC) Foundation Curriculum in 2005, and new post-Foundation specialist training in 2007. The speed with which these changes have been implemented has been bewildering for many trainees and for their trainers. The College decided at an early stage that it would provide enhanced support to trainees to help them navigate through their training within these new systems.

Foundation training is a daunting start to your postgraduate career, and your performance within it will play a major part in your selection for specialist training. Whilst there will no doubt be excellent local support for your learning, we know from more than 15 years of delivering courses and programmes that trainees have widely differing learning requirements and preferences. Some will need extra help with certain aspects of the Foundation Curriculum, whilst others will be looking for more detail in certain topic areas. Your F1 and F2 posts should provide a rich variety of clinical experience to bring your theoretical learning alive. However you will not be able to cover every possible clinical scenario – *STEP^{TM} Foundation* will help cover many of those gaps with scenarios and simulation.

Foundation training is a vital first stage in postgraduate training to which *STEP^{TM} Foundation* offers a unique contribution. It combines tried and tested learning materials and methods developed and updated over a decade and a half, with new material specially written to the Foundation level. *STEP^{TM} Foundation* will act as a bridge, taking you confidently from generic F1 and F2 training to ST1 (Specialist Training Level 1) in surgery or a 'surgically related discipline'.

Mike Larvin, Series Editor

Contributors

Series editor

Professor M. Larvin, Medical School, University of Nottingham, Derby

STEP™ project team

S. Ahmed, Development Editor

D. Atkins, Publications Manager

T. Kamal, Project Coordinator

A. Swales, Project Manager

Authors: Module 1

Mrs H. Allan, The Royal College of Surgeons of England, London

Dr T. N. Appleyard, Northern General Hospital, Sheffield

Dr D. Bryden, Northern General hospital, Sheffield

Dr N. D. Edwards, Northern General Hospital, Sheffield

Dr S. Fletcher, Norfolk & Norwich University Hospital, Norwich

Dr G. W. G. French*, Northampton General Hospital, Northampton

Dr J. B. Groves, Chesterfield & North Derbyshire Royal Hospital, Chesterfield

Mr G. Howell, Scarborough General Hospital, Scarborough

Dr D. Howlett, Eastbourne District General Hospital, Eastbourne

Dr R. Lane, Leeds General Infirmary, Leeds

Professor M. Larvin, Medical School, University of Nottingham, Derby

Mr J. MacFie, Scarborough General Hospital, Scarborough

Mrs J. Murfitt, The Royal College of Surgeons of England, London

Mr J. W. R. Peyton*, Craigavon Area Hospital, Craigavon

Dr R. E. Webster*, Northampton General Hospital, Northampton

We would like to thank all the previous authors, convenors, editors, reviewers, the editorial board and the advisory board for their support and valuable inputs.

Reviewers: Module 1

Mr L. Cascarini, Mr J. W. R. Peyton*, Dr R. E. Webster*

Editorial board

Mr A. J. Brooks*, Dr G. W. G. French*, Miss L. Haine, Dr D. Howlett, Mr M. D. Humzah, Mrs T. Knight, Professor D. G. Lowe, Mr S. J. E. Matthews, Dr Z. T. Maung, Professor K. Mokbel*, Mrs J. Murfitt, Dr K. E. Orr*, Mr M. H. Patterson, Mr J. W. R. Peyton*, Mr N. I. Ramus*, Dr J. R. Stoneham*, Dr R. E. Webster*, Mr D. C. Wilkins

Advisory board

Mrs H. Allan, Mr L. Cascarini, Mrs L. M. de Cossart, Miss L. Haine, Professor N. Horrocks, Professor R. M. Kirk, Professor The Lord McColl, Mrs J. Murfitt, Mr M. H. Patterson, Mr R. C. G. Russell, Mr M. P. Saunders, Mr W. E. G. Thomas

* Convenors of modules.

Acknowledgements

I am greatly indebted to all those formally named in the acknowledgements section. I would also like to offer thanks to the special people who supported me closely in a project, keeping up to the rapid pace required:

The College Council: The council, under its previous president, the late Hugh Phillips, and our current President, Bernard Ribeiro, had the foresight to commit to providing better learning support for trainees, as immense changes in Foundation and specialist surgical training emerged.

The Raven Department of Education: Alan Swales and Natalie Briggs ensured that the project saw the light of day, stuck to deadlines, and smoothed the way to the final production.

College Library: Thalia Knight, Tom Bishop and Polly Setterfield continued to provide great support for STEP™, with online resources for the eSTEP™ Foundation website, reference updates and some great ideas.

The STEP™ project team: Tayyaba Kamal and Judy Murfitt, who have provided me with unswerving support since the launch of eSTEP™ in 2001, and subsequently with STEP™ and the Foundation edition. Tayyaba conducted initial market research and commenced editorial work. Mr Dalvi Humzah took over from me as STEP™ Tutor, and has also developed an innovative and fresh looking eSTEP™ Foundation website, as well as assisting greatly with the project in general.

Editorial team: We received considerable additional editorial support from David Howlett, Professor Jerry Kirk, Kathy Orr, Rodney Peyton, John Stoneham and Rae Webster.

Our two trainee members, Louise Haine and Luke Cascarini, also both provided great assistance. I'm also grateful to Louise for conducting the trainee focus group research.

Publishing: Shehnaz Ahmed carried out all of the vital work required for the editorial management and in-house production of the print material, applying her enormous enthusiasm and great talent. She was ably supported by David Atkins, whose considerable experience in the publishing world resulted in a highly polished final product.

Colleagues: Sue Rougeolle, my Academic PA at the University of Nottingham kept me on the straight and narrow throughout. Many colleagues across the specialties, junior and senior, in the Derby Hospitals Foundation Trust and the Medical School, dealt calmly with numerous queries.

I would also like to pay tribute to the generosity of the late Mrs Maude Guyatt and the late Mr Phillip Cutner FRCS whose generous legacies to the College in large part helped to finance this important project.

Finally I must thank my wife Keyna and our children for their love and patience whilst I wrestled with STEP™ on my laptop at home, on car journeys, during holidays and in many other places.

Mike Larvin

STEP™ Foundation outline

Authors

H. Allan

J. Murfitt

Introduction

Welcome to the distance learning programme—STEP™ Foundation. STEP™ is the Surgical Education and Training Programme of The Royal College of Surgeons of England, and has been in existence since 1994. Distance learning programmes are designed to complement workplace learning. Changes in the way trainees work means that it has assumed even greater importance. Shortened training and reduced hours have improved working lives for trainees, but have reduced the opportunities for learning through experience. This is why your Deanery Foundation programme provides more formal teaching sessions and assessments than previously was the case, both in F1 and F2. There is still a considerable amount of personal learning that you will need to complete in your private study time or during gaps in the working day. Too often students defer their reading instead of immediately resolving a problem or checking it, especially when dealing with clinical problems. We all know knowledge is best remembered when it is linked to a person or patient. Making such links during your day can be invaluable.

STEP™ Foundation aims to support your learning using full colour reading material, containing interactive learning exercises and clinical cases. This is linked to our online support, the eSTEP™ Foundation website, accessible only to STEP™ Foundation registered trainees. You will also receive discounts on the Preparation for Intercollegiate MRCS (IMRCS) Oral Examination and Scientific Basis of Surgical Practice (SBSP) courses administered by The Royal College of Surgeons of England, and on books from partners of STEP™ Foundation, as well as access to the College's extensive library resources (normally only available to members and fellows). Trainees will also be invited to a College induction to explore whether specialist surgical training is the right career choice after Foundation training. We have designed the programme so it covers all the important expected learning outcomes of the Foundation curriculum, as well as testing your progress and advising you on how to proceed.

We start with some guidance on how to get the best out of STEP™ Foundation and then will focus on the main topic of Module 1: Planned Care including elective surgery. Further units in Module 1 will cover communication with patients, legal problems, and the preparation of patients undergoing planned care. Module 2 covers post-procedural care and evidence-based medicine. Topics within these units are mapped to the expected learning outcomes and competences for the F1 year. On completion of F1 you should be able to recognize and deal successfully with most common or routine clinical and related non-clinical situations.

Work through the programme steadily, and we hope that you will enjoy all that it has to offer you at this exciting time of your career!

The STEP™ Team, August 2006

STEP™ Foundation user guide (Please read this first)

STEP™ Foundation is a comprehensive distance learning programme. This module is NOT a textbook, but rather a guide to the comprehensive STEP™ Foundation study programme. Modules use interactive learning exercises and clinical case questions that will help ensure that you not only assimilate new knowledge, but also ensure that you understand it fully and commit it to long-term memory. Work steadily and identify topics that require more work—use a highlighter if you wish, and scribble notes and comments in the wide margins provided. Add links to other useful resources you discover. This will all help you to revise later.

For efficient study, use the blank boxes at the end of each section to mark a tick, writing a date alongside. This will remind you when you have:

- **C** Completed your reading
- **S** Self-assessed using *e*STEP™ Foundation website
- **R** Revised

An example is provided below:

C ☑ *12/08/06*

S ☑ *14/09/06*

R ☑ *13/10/06*

Do remember to log in to *e*STEP™ Foundation regularly. *e*STEP™ Foundation contains a rich variety of supporting material to make your study more efficient. *e*STEP™ Foundation is updated frequently and will contain late-breaking amendments, unit by unit, as well as valuable additional resources.

You will notice four main icons that appear from time to time within the margins. These direct you to reference articles in SURGERY journal, to additional textbook reading, carefully selected weblinks, and to special *e*STEP™ Foundation resources. When you see an icon within a section, you will be able to locate the linked material on *e*STEP™ Foundation by referencing the Module and Unit. The keys to the four Icons are shown below:

 Surgery journal

 eSTEP™ resource

 Textbook

 Weblink

We hope you enjoy working through this Unit. Please use *e*STEP™ Foundation to provide us with your feedback and any comments or suggestions.

Expected learning outcomes

When you have completed this Unit, you will be able to:

- use the learning theory to maximize efficiency of your own studies
- relate learning theory to your own clinical practice
- recognize the cyclical nature of learning and the value of reflective practice
- plan the best use of your precious study time
- set your own learning goals.

Taking your first STEP

EXPERIENTIAL LEARNING

Activists

Reflectors

Theorists

Pragmatists

GETTING THE BEST FROM YOUR STUDY TIME

Taking ownership

Planning

Set your goals

Time management

Little and often

HOW TO APPROACH STEP™ FOUNDATION

Colleagues

Learning as a process of distillation

Note taking—keeping a learning record

Re-evaluation—a review process

Breaking it up

Revision

Last-minute revision

INTEGRATING STEP™ FOUNDATION AND CLINICAL LEARNING

Taking your first STEP

After the constrained environment of your Medical School, the early years of post-graduate medical training must seem daunting, especially at this time of major change in the way it is delivered and assessed. STEP™ Foundation is not a short-cut to learning but, properly used, it will assist you to achieve the fundamental learning goals of the Foundation programme as well as prepare you for the specialist training that follows. STEP™ Foundation not only provides a rich package of learning materials, but also offers you personal learning support which is designed to help you achieve your goals.

Source: www.CartoonStock.com

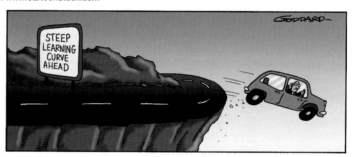

We are all aware of the many demands you have on your time and energy as a newly qualified doctor, so we have tried to make STEP™ Foundation as relevant to the Foundation Curriculum as possible—whether or not you subsequently enter surgical training. As STEP™ Foundation is closely mapped to the Foundation Curriculum it will support your learning throughout F1 and F2 years, as well as allowing you to explore your commitment to specialist surgical training and assist in the next steps towards this if it is your chosen goal.

Doctors (and especially surgeons) demonstrate their professionalism through their ability to think on their feet in stressful situations and to apply principles based on professional knowledge in unknown situations. To be able to do this, you will need to integrate what you learn from STEP™ Foundation with the knowledge and skills you gain from clinical experience and other learning opportunities. These will include your local Trust and Deanery Foundation teaching programme, as well as courses offered by The Royal College of Surgeons of England and the other Royal Colleges in the UK and Ireland. You will need to make the connections between these for yourself, and should seek help from your clinical and educational supervisors, mentors and colleagues.

To get the most out of STEP™ Foundation, it would be best to establish a study routine where you set aside regular time and steadily work through the modules and online activities. You should also take full advantage of the materials available on eSTEP™ Foundation as these are integral to the programme as a whole and complement the printed materials. You will receive advice on how to do this best later in this unit.

This introductory section is divided into three parts:

1 The first part looks at the learning theory behind much of the medical education system, and provides you with a hands-on approach to discovering your own individual learning style and how to harness that knowledge to your best advantage.

2   The second part of this section looks at how you can get the best out of your learning programme. It considers optimal approaches to studying with the STEP™ Foundation materials.

3   The third part addresses the skill of integrating theory (STEP™ Foundation and other learning materials) with practice in your every day clinical experiences.

This is intended to be only a brief guide to help you to manage your training at this early stage in your postgraduate career and to get the most out of every learning situation you find yourself in. It may also help you to decide whether specialist surgical training is the correct career choice for you. Further learning support is always available to you through the *e*STEP™ Foundation learning support area.

Experiential learning

Much of the philosophy underpinning current beliefs on how we learn is derived from the notion of 'Experiential learning', first advanced by the American educationist David Kolb in 1984. It is widely recognized within the medical world that experience underpins all learning and that the search for meaning from experience is fundamental to learning. Learning is concerned with creating meanings and making sense of experiences and this is a process that comes fairly naturally to adults. However, we can maximize our skills in this area by understanding the concepts behind Experiential learning, and also by exploring our own individual learning preferences within the Experiential learning cycle.

This cycle is built around four key aspects of learning:

1   the **practice** in which we are engaged;

2   **reflection** upon that practice;

3   the development of **theoretical** principles from this reflection;

4   the testing, or active **experimentation**, of the theories in practice.

Fig. 1.1.1
The cycle of continuous learning

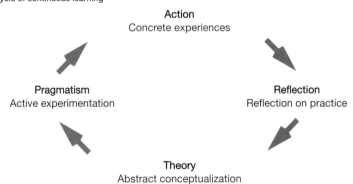

These aspects occur in the Experiential learning cycle and occur in a specific order (Fig. 1.1.1). However, there is no real starting point to the cycle; learning can occur in a cyclical, progressive fashion from any one of the parts of the cycle. So action is not the final end-point of learning, but just one of the many stages through which we and our practice go, in pursuit of improvement and mastery. An amendment to action may be proof that some learning has taken place, but equally we can engage in the learning cycle and decide not to change our actions as a result of our reflections, theorizing and experimentation.

Most of us will be aware of all of the components in this learning cycle and for many of us there will be a preferred area or two within it. You may have noticed from group teaching you have been involved in that learners have different preferences and aptitudes for learning. You may even recognize your own preferences within the following learning styles:

Activists

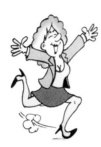

Activists often thrive upon *concrete experiences*, live in the 'here and now' and tend to immerse themselves fully and openly in new experiences. They 'learn by doing'—the traditional surgical learning mode and enjoy participating in group work especially, if they can hog the limelight! They tend to be 'quick fire' when involved in *e*STEP™ Foundation online discussions. They may become bored with very routine activities.

Activists *learn* best in new situations or problems, in games or group work or role play, chairing meetings and discussions. They *learn less well* with lectures, reading or writing alone, absorbing data, following precise instructions.

Reflectors

Reflectors enjoy observing others and *reflecting on practice* from a variety of viewpoints. They like to collect data and analyse, but may be put off coming to solid conclusions. They enjoy problem-based approaches to learning such as provided on *e*STEP™ Foundation but prefer to watch or listen to others before joining in themselves. Watching from the sidelines is not a traditional learning mode for surgeons, but it is an important behaviour to foster in appropriate circumstances. In *e*STEP™ Foundation online discussions they would prefer to think about their response carefully before posting.

Reflectors *learn* best when observing others at work, when they have had time to think about what they have seen, and producing work without tight deadlines. They *learn less* well when asked to lead others, or when role-playing, when they do not have time to prepare, being given very difficult tasks especially when given tight deadlines.

Theorists

Theorists: enjoy forming *abstract concepts*, and try to create ideas that integrate their observations into logical theories to be tested in a step by step way. They tend to be perfectionists and detached rather than emotional. Great surgical pioneers are often theorists in their learning, and although it is not a skill traditionally shared by all surgeons, we need theorists to help move things forward. In *e*STEP™ Foundation online discussions these are the posters who ask searching questions beyond the obvious.

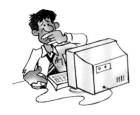

Theorists *learn* best when in difficult situations and they have to draw on their own experiences and skills, when they know exactly what is required of them, and when they have time to think about what they are doing and things not necessarily directly related to it. They *learn less well* when dealing mainly with feelings and emotions, when they are not given a structure to work within, and when they feel out-of-tune with people with other learning styles.

Pragmatists

Pragmatists enjoy *active experimentation* and trying to apply relevant theories to their decision-making and problem-solving processes. They do not enjoy long discussions. Traditionally most surgeons enjoy this approach to learning, as they do in their surgical practice. Pragmatists tend to really enjoy STEP™ Foundation interactive learning exercises.

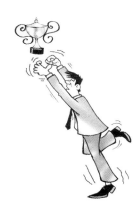

Pragmatists *learn best* when their learning is closely linked to their work, when they can obtain feedback on their learning, for example by role-play, when there are obvious advantages by time saving, and when they are shown a model they can copy. They *learn less well* when learning is largely theoretical, when they cannot recognize any immediate benefit and when there are no guidelines to direct their learning.

Most of us will recognize a little of ourselves in each domain, but one or two will predominate and others will be less applicable to our learning. You can now appreciate why STEP™ Foundation does not rely on a single medium and incorporates both print materials and online resources.

In 1982 Peter Honey and Alan Mumford, two British Educationists, developed a questionnaire to enable learners to identify their strongest and weakest learning preferences. By taking the questionnaire it allows us as learners to build upon strengths and also work to develop the parts of the learning cycle which are less strong, so improving the efficiency of our learning. By doing so you will make your learning easier, more efficient and hopefully more enjoyable. Without it learning may be a random 'hit-and-miss' activity, when what you really need at this stage in your career is far more hits than misses. Knowledge of your learning styles profile allows you to expand your learning experiences and become a more versatile all-rounder. You will learn how to obtain the best learning out of all of the various opportunities arising at work and in your own time, planned and serendipitous. You will become better at self-scrutiny and at making improvements to your learning. Learning to learn more effectively is an important skill!

We would strongly encourage you to take the Honey and Mumford's Learning Styles Questionnaire yourself and look at the analysis and discover what kind of a learner you are. Details of how to do this can be found on the *e*STEP™ Foundation learning support area.

Getting the best from your study time

A plethora of good medical textbooks is now available, as are books that tell you how to study, but in the medical field you face the especial challenge of integrating *what you read* with *what you see and do*: the theory/practice relationship is fundamental to your learning. Building on the experiential learning cycle above, in which you engage in *reflective practice*, here are some guidelines to help you address your study needs as you commence STEP™ Foundation.

The Lumley Study Centre at The Royal College of Surgeons of England. Source: The Royal College of Surgeons of England Photographic Unit

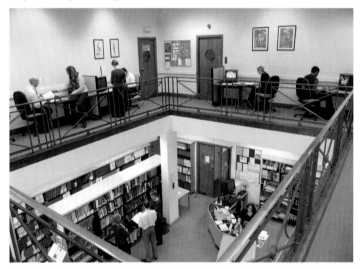

Taking ownership

Learning should never feel like something that has been externally imposed upon you, and so one of the main requirements of you at the outset is that *you take ownership of your learning*. You need to control it, plan for it, organize it, engage in it, relate it to your practical environment and evaluate it.

- Find somewhere physically suitable to study.
- Make sure it is comfortable, warm, light and quiet.
- Make sure you have all the resources and equipment you need.
- Develop a realistic time frame.

Planning

It is critical to get the planning stage right if you are to study well. The memory is like a complex series of boxes. To retain the most information in the most meaningful ways, we have to attach each piece of information to a previously held piece of information—that is, located within the correct box. So planning your study is not just about timetables and comfortable chairs (although they too are important), it is about ensuring that you are able to access and store knowledge which is meaningful to you and your context. This is often called 'meaning making', and if you are to retain lots of new information, you need to make it mean something to you. So plan your learning accordingly:

- Develop a 'discipline map': a plan that provides you with an overview of the areas, principles and concepts that you are expected to learn, as informed by published curricula such as that provided for Foundation training. This will help to structure your mind, guide your learning and organize your time.

● The discipline map can be refined into a more detailed 'road map' which is like a timetable that maximizes your individual areas of learning and experience. You may like to consult your tutor or mentor about this to check you are on the right track.

Set your goals

Ensure that you know the perimeters of the learning session. Do not say to yourself, 'I am going to read as much as I can before I fall asleep.' Rather, tell yourself, 'I have two hours to cover this small section of the workbook. Reading it may take around 40 minutes and the rest of the time I will be making sense of it, note taking, relating it to previous and relevant knowledge, and linking it to what I have experienced in practice.' In this way you are setting meaningful, achievable goals for yourself and giving yourself much more chance to actually master the topic.

Time management

Source: www.CartoonStock.com

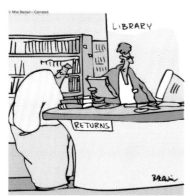

"'Principles of Time Management' was due back six months ago."

Time management's biggest ally is planning. If you plan realistically from the very beginning, and of course, stick to your plan, then your time will not run away with you. It used to be said that you had to study for 20 hours per week for a year (approximately 1000 hours) if you were to pass Part 1 (the Primary) of the old FRCS examination in your first attempt. The new MRCS examination will be much more closely linked to your everyday clinical experience and this should make it easier to see the relationships between the different parts of your training and the examination.

This is why you should keep a record of your learning in order to integrate these differing aspects of your training. You should also spread out your study: 15 hours a week over one year is much more effective than 168 hours a week in the last few weeks. Six days solid with no sleep immediately before the exam will not work! Trainees often tell us (in our surveys) that after they have worked, cooked and cleaned, and attended to all their other responsibilities, there is little time left in their lives for study. Social lives may well have to become dim and distant memories, but if you really target your studying and make sure you learn in the very best possible way for you, this time will be time well spent. Half-hearted studying never pays off. Try to see your study time like money—if you borrow against it, you do need to pay it back again. There are no free gifts and very few loans when you are studying for your professional future.

Little and often

Cramming only works when it is revision of what is already known and properly understood. You cannot input new, meaningful information in the last 72 hours before the examination. You can review what is already known and that is what your final week or two is all about. Studying should take place frequently, for fairly short periods at a time. Whether you set aside 2 hours each day, or choose to cover 14 hours in your day off is up to you. What is important is that you find a way to record and review your learning from both STEP™ Foundation and from your clinical practice, preferably every day, in order to really integrate the different types of learning in which you are engaged. Advice on keeping a learning record is included later.

How to approach STEP™ Foundation

Remember that the programme has been carefully ordered and categorized. We suggest that you start working through the programme module by module, unit by unit, section by section. However we appreciate that you may well want to work ahead and take advantage of the learning opportunities your various Foundation programme posts offer. Modules 1 and 2 cover aspects of routine or planned patient care, mainly to meet the needs of F1 trainees. Module 3 includes the care of acutely ill patients and is suited to F2 trainees. Module 4 covers practical procedures for both F1 and F2, and provides a basic introduction to surgical knowledge at a level appropriate to the first two parts of the planned new-style MRCS examination. Each module is written as a series of units, which are split into sequences of topic sections colour coded in the margins as Basic Sciences or Clinical Topics. Basic Science sections often prepare for subsequent Clinical Topics later in a unit.

Each unit is prefaced by a short introduction and the STEP™ Foundation user guide, an outline of the topics to be covered, and your expected learning outcomes mapped to the Foundation curriculum. Each unit ends with a succinct summary. Most topic sections contain short sections of didactic material, punctuated by Learning exercises, which are designed to probe your existing knowledge and 'make you think'. This approach encourages you to understand what is being taught rather than simply learning facts by rote. The answers are located at least a page or two later, and you will often find the answers a good source of further learning. Scattered throughout the sections are also illustrative clinical cases based on the topic discussed above. If you consistently find you can give all of the correct responses to these two types of in-text questions for a particular topic, then you should move onto self-assessment which is located wholly within the eSTEP™ Foundation website so that we can keep it fully up to date.

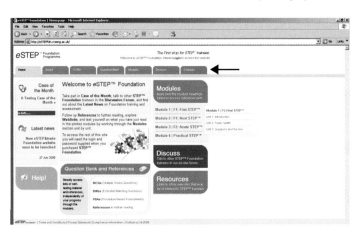

The figure above shows the eSTEP™ Foundation home page at the time of publication (we will continue to update and improve the site, and details may change). To login to the website, use the Athens account details you were given when you purchased STEP™ Foundation.

Navigation around the site is intuitive, but there are also tabs at the top of the page to guide you. The printed modules and the eSTEP™ Foundation website complement each other so when you read the modules, you will see several icons representing resources on this site. For example, if you come across the weblink reference in a topic, go to the eSTEP™ Foundation 'Module Resources' section, 'hover' over the Module and click on the Unit. You will then see the topics for that unit, and you can click on the relevant weblink icon to display the weblink reference that you need. Similarly, you can find self-testing material by clicking on the eSTEP™ Foundation icon at the relevant Unit level.

There are also other resources such as a discussion forum for you to contact us or talk to each other as we know that some trainees can be isolated in their training and we wish to support you. Should you experience any difficulties or have any queries, please contact the STEP™ team whose contact details are on the Contacts tab.

Colleagues

Make sure that senior colleagues in your team know that you are studying using STEP™ Foundation. Although your consultants and seniors may be familiar with the programme, it is a new edition and the first time it has been produced for pre-surgical training. Some of your consultants will have the experience of being examiners for the College, convenors or faculty on College courses, or may even be among our many contributing authors to STEP™ Foundation. You may well find that a senior colleague has studied an earlier version of STEP™, and so will understand the kind of programme you are involved with. Do ask your seniors for advice and help regularly. Choose your moment of course. It is clearly not wise to ask for a chat when the aortic clamp accidentally becomes detached. Suitable moments may include those breaks between operations, allowing for time to write operative notes, or when winding down at the end of clinic.

Good teachers will always make time for their trainees, however busy they are themselves. Find out who the good teachers are in your hospital by asking other trainees. Even if your consultants are not familiar with the STEP™ Foundation edition, they will have been through similar training themselves in the past, and have also worked hard to prepare for post-graduate examinations whether they are surgeons or not. They may provide answers to questions where you do not understand the material, and may also be able to 'test' you informally on anything from anatomy to communication skills. *DO* expect to be quizzed on anatomy in the operating theatre, endoscopy suite and radiology meeting, physiology on the ITU and ward rounds, and pathology at the histology meeting—and *DO* prepare for these events the night before by completing some reading. If you show an interest in your learning in this way you will greatly encourage your seniors to invest their time in assisting you to the best of their abilities. If all else fails or you are attached to a different specialty and cannot get the answer you need, make a posting to the eSTEP™ Foundation learning support service, which can be done anonymously.

Learning as a process of distillation

In accessing, storing and retrieving information, our brains need to process it: distilling, separating and purifying our knowledge to make meaning. It is not enough in today's world to merely regurgitate facts or theories; we need to be able to apply these in practice and show that they have practical meaning for us. So a special kind of note taking is required.

Note taking—keeping a learning record

Copying out the syllabus (defined as a list of topics which will be assessed in an examination) is no longer enough. You need to develop a way to make meaning between what you read, what you see and what you do. A very useful way to do this is to create a record of some sort. In other areas of learning this may be called a Learning Journal: a record of what has been seen, read, heard and done with a commentary which links to previous knowledge or skills. This is one way of making sense of all of your experiences. If you are to distil all of this into meaningful and, more importantly, retrievable knowledge you must find a way of refining and reducing it and this is where regular review is very useful.

Across the STEP™ Foundation printed material you will find wide margins designed to encourage you to make notes about your learning. Use the various tick boxes to show which pages you have read, self-assessed and revised and, ideally, note the dates—this will greatly assist at revision time! Tick off or ring the various links to *e*STEP™ Foundation and weblinks to carefully selected external online resources, and also investigate the references to textbooks and Surgery journal. In some instances, you may feel you already know a lot about the topic and can skip some of the links—you do not have to follow them all. The links are there to tell you what extra material is available. Log onto *e*STEP™ Foundation regularly, and you will remember that Athens password when you really feel the need to use the site during revision periods.

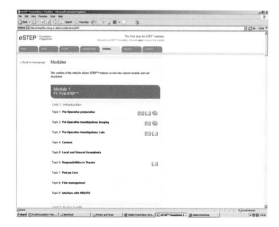

Re-evaluation—a review process

When accessing and storing information, it is good to engage in a process of evaluation and re-evaluation. We evaluate new information by considering its use to us: is it information we need to have? If it is, we then re-evaluate our experience in the light of this information. There are four aspects of re-evaluation which can enhance reflection and individual learning.

1 Association: relating new ideas to those already known.
2 Integration: seeking relationships between old and new.
3 Validation: determining the relevance of these ideas.
4 Appropriation: making the knowledge our own.

By following this approach, perhaps again by scribbling in the margins, you can successfully refine and reduce your information store into that which is meaningful and relevant to you.

Breaking it up

Reading, note taking and keeping a learning journal are excellent ways of making meaning, but they are lengthy. How can you remember all you need to remember come exam time? You need to build into your study regime a regular review process whereby you look over your notes, refine them and focus on the areas with which you are not yet familiar. If this is done regularly, once a week perhaps, it will ensure that more information is stored and so there is less panic in those precious weeks before the exam.

Revision

The materials for this programme have been designed so that you can begin to plan your revision programme from day 1. Use the tick boxes to show what you have done or not, write notes in the margins, and together with your personal notes and learning record you will gradually build up your own totally individual revision pack which suits the way you learn best. If you choose to keep a learning record, then look at this regularly, especially when revising for the exam.

Last-minute revision

This should really not involve any new material—leave time to ensure that your reading is complete before you start revising! In the last two weeks, maybe more, before an assessment, 'retrieval' should be the main objective. Ask yourself, 'Can I remember all I need to about this topic?' All of the information inputting and storing should already have been done. You are now sorting through your memory to organize the knowledge for quickest and best retrieval.

Integrating STEP™ Foundation and clinical learning

Making sense of the relationship between theory and practice requires you to engage in organized reflective learning before you implement what you have learned in your everyday work. You need to ensure that you can access, store and retrieve information and experiences that are meaningful and relevant to your learning. Support in this area will be extremely varied according to your location and the context in which you work so it is very important that you take control of your own learning so that it is meaningful and relevant to you.

There will be many opportunities for you to integrate what you have been reading in the STEP™ Foundation materials with what you see, hear and do in your clinical practice. In ward rounds, clinics, theatre and small group work you will have plenty of opportunities to test out or analyse your theoretical knowledge in the context of practical patient care. If STEP™ Foundation is to be meaningful and relevant to your life as a junior doctor you need to develop the skills of integrating theory (learning materials) with practice (your clinical life). Here are some of the ways in which you can maximize this theory–practice relationship and ensure you are getting the most out of your experiences.

An Intercollegiate Basic Surgical Skills (BSS) course in progress at The Royal College of Surgeons of England. Source: The Royal College of Surgeons of England Photographic Unit

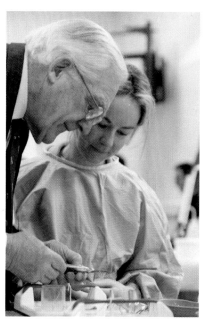

You can learn just as effectively from others as from your own experiences: Even when you are not directly involved in a clinical exercise, you can use it to reflect upon what you have read, what others are saying, what you are seeing of the patient, or hearing from the consultant or registrar leading the group.

Record what you see and do on a daily basis: Cases do not occur in a sensible or logical order and many good trainers will take advantage of opportunistic learning in clinical settings. Because the clinical training may not always occur in a logical and syllabus-like sequence, you will have to take care to record what you have learned each day and tie it into your STEP™ Foundation-based learning activities. This is where a learning record is useful.

Review your existing knowledge: Whenever you are in a clinical setting and are learning from that setting, remember to file the new knowledge away with the relevant existing knowledge you have—it will make for better retention of the topic.

Identify goals for yourself: Goals may not always be made explicit in the clinical setting, especially when working under pressure or opportunistically. It is important that in order for you to retain the new learning in which you are engaged, you are able to identify the goals of the learning session. This will make it clearer for you to see what the session is about and where it fits overall with STEP™ Foundation.

Interact with colleagues: Ask questions if you are unsure. If it is not possible for you to ask questions during the session, then find someone to ask afterwards. Do not allow yourself to go away with misconceptions. Also, do not be afraid to question your colleagues if there is a discrepancy between what you have covered in STEP™ Foundation, and what you have seen or been told in the clinical context. Use *e*STEP™ Foundation for those questions you do not feel able to ask colleagues; you can post them anonymously if you so wish!

Feedback: *DO* seek feedback. This is not just on practical matters such as performing a clinical skill, but do seek feedback on your progress as a whole, on your study approach, especially with a colleague who is familiar with STEP™ Foundation, even if this is from previous editions. Managing your learning is almost as big a job as actually learning. If learning is not organized, well planned, regularly engaged in and reviewed both by yourself and by others, then it is not necessarily being most effective.

The formal teaching round: Teaching rounds tend to be formal episodes with specific time set aside for the study of an isolated case or number of cases. There may well be the opportunity for you to plan in advance and so *do* read the relevant parts of STEP™ Foundation edition. Often the disease process is the central theme with history taking and clinical examination being the starting points for discussion. The teaching tends to be theoretically based and will often complement STEP™ Foundation materials. However, with the emphasis on theory, this is a good opportunity for you to relate ideas to practice and to ask questions about the practical and clinical issues surrounding the topic.

The ward round: 'Teaching' ward rounds often have little opportunity for students to contribute and you are more likely to be on the receiving end of low-level questions from the trainer. This does not mean that they are not valuable areas of learning. Once again, make sure you record and review what you have seen and discussed and review the relevant areas of STEP™ Foundation materials too. Remember, this learning process is your own responsibility.

Identify your needs and concerns: Because you are largely responsible for your progress through this stage of your training, especially with regard to STEP™ Foundation, you need to ensure that if and when you have worries and concerns you find some way of both identifying them and seeking help with them. You may have been allotted a mentor or a designated person to oversee your training. You should have both a programme-based educational supervisor and post-based clinical supervisor. It is important that you meet with both at the specified intervals—this enables them to support you as best as they can. You may also seek out a colleague, a more senior trainee, or consultant who is familiar with your study programme, and willing to assist you in clarifying uncertainties.

Consolidation of learning: One trainee told us, 'revising such a large amount of material is difficult, as there is not enough time to review the whole thing.' This is where reviewing and summarizing is most useful. When you have recorded and reviewed your learning for the day, it may be useful to summarize, perhaps on record cards, what you have covered, and keep these summaries for revision and review purposes in the future. You can look at them to jog your memory not just before the exam but perhaps before you know you are going to be doing some clinical work in that area. Regular review of your records will ensure that the knowledge is firmly filed away in your brain, ready for access at any time.

Summary

In this Unit you have studied the need for direction in your Foundation programme learning, and have learned what being an adult, professional learner means. We have discussed the importance of modern learning theory and how it can increase the efficiency of your learning activities. You should also now appreciate the importance of theory and how it must be related to clinical practice. You now recognize the cyclical nature of learning and how valuable reflective practice can be for learning. Above all, you have learned about the importance of planning the best use of your precious study time, and have become determined to set appropriate learning goals. If you would like to find out more about effective learning, please go to the *e*STEP™ Foundation website resources.

Comments from previous trainees about STEP™

In the assessment you have to marshal your thoughts in a coherent way. STEP™ gives you the knowledge of the subjects and you can use the STEP™ self-assessment to check your understanding. To simulate the stressful conditions of the assessment you should ask colleagues to test you on subjects as they come up in everyday clinical work.

STEP™ is well organized and structured. It teaches you to organize your learning and plan revision.

The material and layout is good, and very colourful which helps with the learning process. I like the questions section and the answers are given in good detail.

Extremely relevant. Added structure to my learning. It helped me organize my study sessions.

Very useful. I like the question and answer approach— it makes you think harder!

The doctor–patient relationship

Authors

R. Lane

R. E. Webster

Introduction

Learning about communication is an appropriate start to the vocational elements of STEP™ Foundation. You should be in no doubt as to the importance of communication, or more correctly, good communication. Good in the sense that what is communicated is appropriate and conveyed with high-fidelity, and good in the sense that it seems satisfactory to our patients. To a frightened patient and their family, good communication is equally as important as a doctor's technical competence, yet far less attention is accorded to it in our training.

The Foundation Curriculum states: 'Doctors must be able to develop, encourage and maintain successful professional relationships with their patients and widely understand the patients' expectations and experience of care; their practice should reflect such understanding.' To do this we must perfect our ability to communicate well. Doctors have varying levels of communication skills, and it is only relatively recently that medical communication has received serious scientific study.

We inhabit a highly specialized world in our work, dealing with complex phenomena and incomplete knowledge, but this world is firmly centred on humanity. To be able to restore an unwell patient to health, we must first extract useful data from patients by careful history taking, weigh it with other data from examination and investigations, formulate diagnoses and further plans, refine this all to recommend appropriate treatments, and of course explain everything and break news along the way—to an appropriate level of understanding for individual patients, their family and friends. Good communication is needed—listening and speaking skills, as well as recognizing the importance of non-verbal communication. It's a tall order!

This Unit should aid your prior understanding of what patients need from you with respect to communication. Module 3 will include further material on communicating with colleagues with seniors, peers and juniors. For the moment, focus on the patient, but bear in mind that many of the skills are generic and can be used with colleagues too. Use your clinical experience to test and improve your personal communications skills. Go and sit in when bad news is broken by your seniors. Take the opportunity to follow the advice in the Foundation Curriculum to seek a formal training course in Communication skills. These allow you to build confidence, especially when they involve the use of actors as simulated patients

This Unit will explore the attitudes, knowledge and skills required to maximize your ability to quickly develop effective and productive relationships with patients. It focuses on the doctor–patient relationship as an equal partnership between two experts.

STEP™ Foundation user guide

Work steadily and identify topics that require more work—use a highlighter if you wish, and scribble notes and comments in the wide margins provided. Add links to other useful resources you discover. This will all help you to revise later.

For efficient study, use the tick boxes at the end of each section, writing a date alongside. This will remind you when you have:

- **C** Completed your reading
- **S** Self-assessed using *e*STEP™ Foundation
- **R** Revised

Do remember to log in to *e*STEP™ Foundation regularly. *e*STEP™ Foundation contains a rich variety of supporting material to make your study more efficient. *e*STEP™ Foundation is updated frequently and will contain late-breaking amendments, unit by unit, as well as valuable additional resources.

 Surgery journal

 eSTEP™ resource

 Textbook

 Weblink

We hope you enjoy working through this Unit. Please use *e*STEP™ Foundation website to provide us with feedback and any comments or suggestions.

Expected learning outcomes

When you have completed this Unit, you will be able to:

- recognize the imbalance in the doctor–patient relationship
- examine the components of emotional intelligence
- apply appropriate communication skills during a consultation to build an effective relationship
- use active listening techniques
- establish empathy between yourself and your patients
- cultivate a patient-centred partnership.

Clinical topics

Clinical topics

Introduction

Source: www.CartoonStock.com

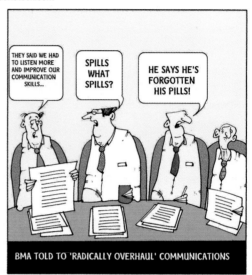

Words are, of course, the most powerful drug used by mankind—Rudyard Kipling

You may have seen this famous quote from a well-known English author before. However perhaps if you think about it carefully you will realise that Kipling got it wrong. Words are very important, but they are not the complete story. The power of the words depends on the context in which they are spoken, and the relationship between the speaker and the recipient is a key determinant of that context. It is essential for you as a doctor to remember this when communicating with any of your patients.

Let's begin with a brief learning exercise to assess how much you remember about what you learned about communication at medical school:

Learning exercise	1

Can you think of all of the different ways that humans use to communicate with?

Learning exercise	2

Can you estimate the relative importance of each of these? To help with this, think about how misunderstandings may arise when communication takes place only by telephone or e-mail.

In the medical consultation it is, to a large extent, the relationship between doctor and patient that shapes how the words are perceived. The doctor–patient relationship is a very unbalanced relationship as both parties have entirely different roles. Both parties can be considered to be experts though. The doctor has more medical knowledge than the patient but the patient is the expert on how their illness or disease is affecting them as an individual.

Fig. 1.2.1

The medical consultation.

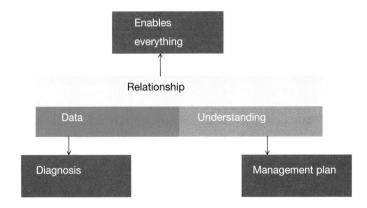

Figure 1.2.1 shows a simplification of the processes operating during a consultation.

Looking at a medical consultation from this viewpoint, you can see that there is a continuous exchange of data (information) between the patient and doctor. This enables the doctor to make a diagnosis or determine which test(s) may be required and also enables the patient to increase their knowledge of their illness.

In a good consultation there is a continuous checking of the understanding of the data exchanged between the doctor and the patient to ensure that they are aware of each other's perspective and that where possible, their understandings of the meaning of the information are the same. The endpoint of such a consultation is to produce a mutually agreed management plan.

A good doctor–patient relationship ensures the doctor's professional integrity is maintained and that the patient feels valued, respected and committed to the management plan.

Remember however that this is an unbalanced relationship. The data exchanged relates solely to the person who has accepted the role of the patient. It would be seen as inappropriate if a doctor gave personal information about their own health to the patient. The doctor is looking at this information in order to make a diagnosis and give the patient what the doctor considers appropriate options to manage the illness or condition of the patient. The patient is looking for expert knowledge and access to treatment for something which is (to a variable extent) disrupting their life. The patient also wants to tell the doctor about the impact the disease or illness is having on all the various aspects of their life.

Learning exercise	3

Can you think of any factor that will hinder the patient feeling that their needs are being met?

Learning exercise	4

When do you think that you might feel you are not giving the patient what they need? Can you think of three issues?

Answers to learning exercises

1. Humans use words to communicate, with modifications to the delivery of these words by the use of tone and volume. They also modify the meaning or emphasis of the words used by adding gestures and other non-verbal behaviour.

2. It may surprise you to know that, in 1981, the Californian psychologist Albert Mehrabian showed that only 7% of communication related to words alone, a further 38% was due to how the words were spoken, but the majority of communication (55%) was due to other factors called body language'.

   This is a very important thing for you to remember. One study demonstrated that when doctors sit down to talk to their patients, the time the doctor is giving to the patient appears to the patient to be longer than when the doctor remains standing. Leaning forward to listen to the patient also has been found to help patients relax, be happier with the outcomes of consultations and remember more of what was discussed.

3. Time is a major factor in this. If you are working in the hospital environment you will have to learn how to establish a rapport with your patients is a very short space of time. They may arrive in A&E or the Emergency Admission Wards as urgent admissions or you may meet them for the first time in an In-patient ward almost immediately prior to an operation. You will not always be on duty, so will have to hand over the care of these patients to another doctor or team. You are also likely to meet a patient for the first time when you are covering for someone else and one of their patients needs some medical attention.

4. Three issues that might affect your ability to give the patient what they need:
   1. Time: As discussed in the last question, you may feel that you never have enough time to actually get to know your patients well enough.
   2. Resources: Easy access to important investigations and the results of these is also not universally available. For example you may have a patient who develops chest pain in the middle of the night three days post-operatively. One of your differential diagnoses would be a pulmonary embolism, but your hospital may not provide an emergency service for the appropriate lung scan to help you in your diagnosis and treatment for this patient.
   3. Uncertainty: Not all illnesses are easy to diagnose or treat. If you are uncertain about a diagnosis or the likely outcome of any treatment you may feel you are not giving your patients what they need from you. Acknowledging uncertainty and its impact on the patient can help the patient cope with and accept levels of uncertainty.

Emotional intelligence

Take care not to make intellect your God—Albert Einstein

You may think that these are strange words for one of the greatest intellects of modern science but Einstein knew that intellect was not everything. This is particularly true when you are considering the processes involved in building a relationship. To build an

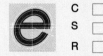

C ☐
S ☐
R ☐

effective relationship, high levels of what is known as 'emotional intelligence' may be required.

Work on emotional intelligence has advanced considerably in the last 20 years. In the book published in 1995, *Emotional intelligence: why it can matter more than IQ*, Goleman, an American psychologist, explored the nature and the importance of emotional intelligence in success. He argued that it contributed more than the type of intelligence which can be measured by IQ tests.

Goleman outlined five components of emotional intelligence as:

1 self-awareness;
2 self-regulation;
3 motivation;
4 empathy;
5 social skills.

Learning exercise	5

Write a sentence to describe what each of these components means to you and think about why they might be considered important factors in establishing relationships.

See answers to learning exercises on page 33.

Skills

The ability of individuals to form effective relationships varies a great deal but luckily for all of us, the required skills can be learned and developed. These skills are behavioural in nature and as such may require different learning techniques to the more usual types of cognitive learning. Behavioural learning usually requires more time, and also the opportunity to practice these behaviours and receive both positive and negative feedback.

Source: www.CartoonStock.com

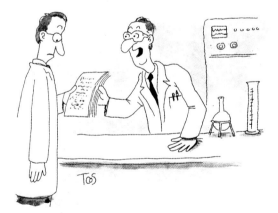

"You've gotta help me! I can't read my own writing!"

The Royal College of General Practitioners has listed the communication and consulting competences required for an effective doctor-patient relationship. These are applicable to all doctors, whatever their chosen specialty.

• Respecting patients as competent and equal partners with different areas of expertise.

- Sharing decision-making with patients, enabling them to make informed choices.
- Respecting patients' perception of the experience of their illness (health beliefs); their social circumstances, habits, behaviour, attitude to risk, values and preferences.
- Understanding the role of patients' ideas, values, concerns and expectations in their understanding of their problems.
- Incorporating patients' expectations, preferences and choices in formulating an appropriate management plan.
- Showing an interest in patients, being attentive to their problems, treating them politely, considerately, and demonstrating active listening skills.
- Demonstrating communication and consultation skills and showing familiarity with well-recognized consultation techniques.
- Establishing effective rapport with the patient.
- Responding to patients' verbal and non-verbal cues to any underlying concerns.
- Being able to detect, elicit and respond to patients' emotional issues.
- Being able to deal with patients' difficult emotions, for example denial, anger, fear.
- Making links between emotional and physical symptoms, or between physical, psychological and social issues.
- Communicating and articulating with patients effectively, clearly, fluently and framing content at an appropriate level, wherever the consultation takes place, including by telephone or in writing.
- Involving patients' significant others such as their next of kin or carer, when appropriate, in a consultation.
- Sensitively minimizing any potentially embarrassing physical or psychological exposure by respecting patients' dignity, privacy and modesty.
- Explaining to the patient the purpose and nature of an examination and offering a chaperone when appropriate.
- Where appropriate, facilitating changes in patients' behaviour.
- Having an understanding of family or group dynamics sufficient to allow effective intervention in patients' family contexts.
- Demonstrating an awareness of the doctor as a therapeutic agent, the impact of transference and counter-transference, the danger of dependency, and displaying an insight into the psychological processes affecting the patient, doctor and relationship between them.
- Understanding the factors, such as longer consultations, which are associated with a range of better patient outcomes.

Calgary–Cambridge Framework

The Calgary–Cambridge Framework was devised by Silverman, Kurtz and Draper in 2005 and describes a framework of the consultation which most closely resembles the realities of medicine.

The framework shows the phases of the consultation moving from initiation of the consultation, gathering information, physical examination, explanation and planning to closure of the session. It is important to remember the two themes that run constantly through every phase—the provision of structure and the building of the relationship. Relationship building is a constant activity from the beginning to the end of the consultation and not an event that occurs at a point in the consultation.

Fig. 1.2.2

The Calgary–Cambridge Framework. From Silverman, Kurtz and Draper (2004). Skills for commmunicating with patients, 2nd edn. page 19. Radcliffe Publishing Ltd.

Initiating the session

- Preparation
- Establishing initial rapport
- Identifying the reason(s) for the consultation

Providing the structure

- Making the organization overt
- Attending to flow

Gathering information

Exploration of the patient's problems to discover the:

☐ biomedical perspective   ☐ patient's perspective

☐ background information: context

Physical examination

Explanation and planning

- Providing the correct amount and type of information
- Aiding accurate recall and understanding
- Achieving a shared understanding incorporating the patient's illness framework
- Planning shared decision-making

Closing the session

- Ensuring appropriate point of closure
- Forward planning

Building the relationship

- Using the appropriate non-verbal behaviour
- Developing a rapport
- Involving the patient

Looking carefully at the framework, now try the next learning exercise:

Learning exercise	6

The authors of the Calgary–Cambridge Framework defined a number of objectives to be accomplished in building a relationship. What do you think they may include?

See answers to learning exercises on page 33.

Of all the skills the doctor must develop, those of building a relationship are among the most important and underpin all other consultation skills. Effective relationship building relies on our attentiveness to the patient as a person and not just a pathological process, our ability to appear 'warm' to the patient and to convey empathy, our willingness to offer emotional support, to show respect for the patient and his or her views and beliefs (even if we do not agree with these views or beliefs), and our willingness and ability to work in partnership with patients.

Attentiveness

Without attentiveness to the patient we are unable to observe the other aspects of the interaction on which we will build to develop a strong doctor-patient relationship—we will not realise when an appropriate opportunity arises to express empathy or to develop partnership working for example. If you are listening carefully to the patient and using appropriate eye contact you are more likely to be able to detect emotional distress. Similarly, greater patient satisfaction has been demonstrated when doctors use appropriate non-verbal communication.

Burnard described 3 zones for attention in 1992:

- Zone 1—attention 'out': focused on the outside world and on the patient
- Zone 2—attention 'in': attention focused on own thoughts and feelings
- Zone 3—attention focused on fantasy

In zone 1 our attention is focused outside of ourselves and we are aware of what the other person is saying and what they are trying to communicate to us.

In zone 2 we focus on our thoughts and feelings relating to the consultation, i.e. how we are reacting to what the patient is communicating. Our own thoughts and feelings give us insights into the patient and are an important part of giving our attention to the patient. Hence it is important that we spend the majority of our time in zone 1 but periodically check our own reactions in zone 2.

In zone 3 we are starting to make assumptions about the patient based on our own beliefs and values, an area Burnard terms fantasy, as we can not know what is being felt or thought by the other person without asking and checking it out. If we focus on zone 3 we run the risk of developing a very distorted picture of our patient and of going on to make further assumptions. The zone of fantasy is best avoided if we want to build open and trusting relationships with patients. It is important that we learn to distinguish between the zone of thinking and feeling and that of fantasy—a key part of the emotional intelligence concept of self-awareness.

A good example of this is if you have had an unsatisfactory appraisal as a trainee. Your appraiser may have told you that others feel you are acting in a certain way and then attempted to tell you why you are doing this. These 'others' are likely to be basing their opinions on their own thoughts and feelings and projecting these onto your behaviour. A much more productive approach would be to tell you what has been observed and ask you if you could explain why you think that might happen.

Active listening

Our attentiveness is conveyed to the patient by active listening. This is much more than just hearing the words.

Fig. 1.2.3

Active listening

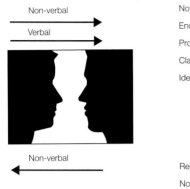

Non-verbal

Verbal

Non-verbal

Noting verbal and non-verbal cues

Encouraging further disclosure

Probing to:

Clarify

Identify

    Missing areas

    Avoided topics

    Feelings, beliefs, concerns, expectations

Responding:

Non-verbal

Verbal

Not only must we give our patient our attention but, to be effective, we must also convey warmth in that attention and ensure that we are not projecting a cold analytical approach. You may not actually be very aware of how you are really seen by your patients. During your career you will be developing a way of appearing as calm as possible in emergency situations (even though inside you are likely to feel very different!). This sometimes extends into the interactions with patients at other times, so that when you think you are conveying feeling, your body language might not be.

Warmth can be conveyed to the patient by touch in the form of an initial handshake or by a comforting touch during the consultation when the patient looks distressed. A posture with the head bent forward indicates attention and concern. Think about your experiences and observations of this.

Learning exercise	7

Can you think of some non-verbal aspects of communication? And non-verbal aspects of speech itself?

See answers to learning exercises on page 33.

The face with its multitude of expressions can convey warmth with a welcoming smile or a look of sadness that tells the patient you understand their concerns. As eye contact is an extremely important non-verbal indicator of attention and concern, it is essential that you maintain this during any communication with your patients. If you are unable to do this, for example if you need to use a computer or write notes, you should explain this to the patient. When eye contact is to be absent it is important that this is not at emotional parts of the consultation and that it is kept to the minimum.

You may be interested to know that a relationship has been shown between the tone of voice used by a surgeon and the frequency that patients make complaints about them.

Empathy

In building an effective relationship the doctor needs to be able to read the patients non-verbal communication and respond appropriately to it. The ability to interpret body language is a key skill that allows the expression of empathy.

Being empathic is one of the strongest factors in building successful professional relationships with patients. Empathy is an attempt to put yourself in the patient's situation and see the world from his or her point of view. This contrasts with sympathy where you express your emotions about the patient's predicament. The work of Maguire and colleagues in 1996 showed that empathy is one of the key skills in helping patients disclose their concerns and it is also a key factor in patient satisfaction with a consultation. The most important aspect of empathy is actually expressing it. Only thinking and feeling it is of no use to the patient. It is the attempt to express empathy that is important; the patient appreciates that you are trying and does not expect you to get it right every time. If, for example, you make a statement like 'I guess that must have been a frightening experience' and you are wrong, the patient will simply correct you by saying, for example, 'No, not really, I was surprised how calm I remained.' Whether you get it right or wrong the attempt to put yourself in the patient's situation helps to build the relationship.

Hence it can be seen that empathy is a two-stage process. First the attempt is to understand the other person and then to express that understanding in a supportive and sensitive way.

Empathy is an excellent way of responding to the patient's emotions. Some doctors may fear that if they encourage their patients to express their emotions, this will in some way be damaging or leave them unable to control the consultation and keep to task. Neither fear is, in fact, correct. Patients find it helpful to be allowed to express their feelings, provided they are not pushed into expressing emotions that they wish to keep private. Again it has been demonstrated that the use of empathy actually makes consultations more efficient.

The communication of empathy is done both verbally and non-verbally. Silverman and colleagues (Calgary–Cambridge Framework) recommended the technique of linking 'I' and 'you' in the empathic sentence, for example:

I guess this is a difficult subject for you.

I can see how upset this has made you.

I can understand how frightened you must be when your pain comes back.

Other key skills that build relationships are acceptance, support, sharing thoughts and providing rationale for what we do. We may not agree with everything our patients tell us but we must respect what they say as a valid opinion or emotion. Using acknowledging responses allows us to value a patient's contribution and prevents us from immediately responding with our own views. In accepting the patient's response we will frequently need to demonstrate this by naming an emotion or summarizing thoughts expressed.

Learning exercise   8

Can you think what is wrong with the following statement?

What I think you are telling me is that you suspect the cough and weight loss are caused by cancer and that this is frightening you, but I can think of many other reasons for your symptoms and don't think you should be worrying yourself.

How could you rephrase the sentence in a more productive way?

Distancing

In 1994, Maguire and Faulkner wrote about 'distancing' by health-care professionals. This is a way of coping with emotionally charged situations or of avoiding continual emotional exposure. You may recognize these tactics from your own practise and in the behaviour which you have witnessed from your colleagues.

What 'distancing techniques' are you aware of?

Answers to learning exercises

5   Self-awareness is seen as the first step towards emotional intelligence. It can be defined as an ability to recognize and understand our own moods, emotions and drives and how they impact others.

Self-regulation is the ability to take control of our emotions, to ensure that negative emotions do not impact on relationships and to redirect our emotions to more positive states that will bring benefit to our interactions.

Motivation requires being able to channel one's emotions to achieve a goal. This often involves deferring gratification until later, and the maintenance of productivity whilst undertaking activities of low interest and pleasure to see a final goal achieved.

Empathy is the action of understanding, being aware of and being sensitive to the feelings of others, despite the fact that these feelings have not been communicated in an explicit way.

Social skills are the set of behaviours that are necessary to establish positive interactions between people who do not know each other well. These include such things as shaking hands when you are first introduced to someone, smiling, listening, being polite and even remembering that you have met someone before!

Being empathic and having social skills are also vitally important in building and managing relationships, especially when it comes to establishing common ground between individuals and managing conflict.

6   Objectives include:

- developing a rapport to enable the patient to feel understood, valued and supported;
- establishing trust between doctor and patient, laying down the foundation for a therapeutic relationship;
- encouraging an environment that maximizes accurate and efficient initiation, information gathering, and explanation and planning;
- enabling supportive counselling as an end in itself;
- developing and maintaining a continuing relationship over time;
- involving the patient so that he or she understands and is comfortable with

participating fully in the process of the consultation;

- reducing potential conflict between doctor and patient;
- increasing both the patient's and the doctor's satisfaction with the consultation.

7   The non-verbal aspects of communication include:

- touch;
- proximity;
- posture;
- physical appearance;
- facial expression and gestures;
- eye contact.

Non-verbal aspects of speech include:

- timing;
- tone;
- errors.

8   You have used the word 'but' and therefore lost the opportunity to allow the patient time to respond to you.

You have acknowledged the patient's views and feelings but then immediately overridden them with your 'superior' knowledge. This not only devalues the patient's contribution but is likely to prevent expansion by the patient.

9   You might say:

What I think you are telling me is that you suspect the cough and weight loss are caused by cancer and that this is frightening you.

This type of response is strengthened by going on to legitimize the patient's response, for example:

I'm glad you mentioned that, it could be important.

10   Easily observed distancing tactics include:

- ignoring cues;
- selective attention to cues: picking up on the physical ones and ignoring the emotional;
- being unrealistically positive particularly when the patient is expressing doubts or concerns, such as often ignoring the patient's expressed concerns;
- normalization of events or feelings;
- premature or false reassurance;
- topic changing;
- passing the buck;
- premature problem solving;
- avoidance of the patient.

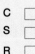

C ☐
S ☐
R ☐

Patient-centred partnership

Try to cultivate the idea of a partnership between you and the patient. This is important as patients wish to be seen as a complete human beings and not just someone who has a particular disease or an illness. When the patient is encouraged to talk about psychosocial issues such as their family or job, the consultation usually only takes a couple of minutes longer, but the patient's satisfaction with the process is improved.

Support can be expressed through overt partnership statements (*I want us to work together in helping you lose weight*), expression of concern (*It worries me that with this degree of pain you will not be able to cope alone over the weekend*), expressions of willingness to help and also by acknowledgement of the efforts our patients have made especially in self-management (*Increasing your painkillers was the right thing to do*).

Sharing our thoughts with our patients and explaining the reasons for what we do, helps us demonstrate our attempts to respect their autonomy.

It is also important to allow the patient to express their worries and opinions by the use of open-ended questions. 'How have you been since the last time I saw you?' is an example of an open-ended question. This has been shown to reduce the frequency of last minute questions by the patient.

Developing patient-centred partnerships and improving your communication skills will have two benefits for you as a doctor. The first is that your job satisfaction will improve and the second is that your patients are less likely to complain against you. If you think about this, these are huge advantages for your working life.

Look at the following cases which have aspects of poor communication and try to decide what went wrong and the reasons for this.

Clinical case 1

Mrs O'Keefe is a 36-year-old married woman with a malignant lump in the left breast. Her GP refers her to a general surgeon, who tells her that she must have a mastectomy. After the operation, the surgeon gives her a cursory explanation of the procedure and leaves the room saying, 'Don't worry, your husband will soon get used to it!' When she attends her follow-up appointment, Mrs O'Keefe is alone, clearly unhappy and angry. She appears embarrassed and will not look at the operation site. She does not have a prosthesis, but has filled her bra with some tissues.

How would you have managed this case differently if she had been your patient?

Q1   At the initial consultation?

Q2   By referring her to other health-care professionals?

Q3   In the clinic at her follow-up appointment?

Clinical case 1 answers

Q1   This surgeon is clearly a poor advertisement for our profession! Mrs O'Keefe required sensitive management and to be treated as an autonomous individual. She is young and faces not only a life-threatening illness but also may feel that the operation itself is a form of mutilation. She should have been given a description of the options available to her and time to talk through these options with the surgeon. Breast cancer is a common disease and she may have a friend or relative who has been affected by this. She will also almost certainly have read a lot about it in the media and on the internet so may be quite well informed already.

Q2 Prior to surgery Mrs O'Keefe should also have been seen by a trained breast counsellor. This would have given her the opportunity to talk about her fears and concerns about her disease and also another opportunity to discuss the various options for treatment and after surgery a prosthesis, albeit temporary, should have been fitted to provide some restoration of normal appearance.

Q3 Her husband should be have been encouraged to attend the follow-up clinic. Any lack of understanding or sympathy from her spouse could then have been detected and discussed. Mrs O'Keefe is likely to feel less physically attractive and may have concealed the operation site completely. She also may be worrying about her husbands feelings about the effects of her disease and her likely prognosis.

You should discuss the situation openly with the patient and her husband and ensure that there is no difficulty with communication between them relating to her physical appearance and the probable effects on her of the rest of her treatment plan and more importantly her likely prognosis.

You should examine the operation site and encourage the patient to look at and touch the area. Use a mirror if necessary. If it is appropriate, you should also discuss reconstructive surgery.

Clinical case 2

A 45-year-old woman, Tania Turner, is admitted to hospital with epigastric pain. The surgical registrar informed her that she has a gastric ulcer discovered during a barium meal which her GP had arranged and which had been done a week before her admission. The registrar had also mentioned the possibility of some ulcers being 'dangerous' and suggested an endoscopy. The patient's father had died of carcinoma of the stomach, but, as the trainee who clerked her in did not ask any questions about her family history, none of the team looking after her in the ward were aware of this. On the consultant's ward round, the registrar presented the case and a discussion took place at the end of the bed. There was a debate between the consultant and the trainee surgeons about whether or not endoscopy should be done, or whether the patient should be scheduled for an immediate laparotomy and gastrectomy. It seemed to Tania that this latter approach was clearly the consultant's choice. She agreed to have a laparotomy and this was done later on the day of her admission. At surgery an antral lesion was found with no obvious spread, and a Billroth I gastrectomy was performed.

Subsequent histology showed a benign gastric ulcer although there was some cellular atypia at the edge of the ulcer and the histopathologist recommended endoscopic follow-up of this. Tania was constantly asking the nursing and medical staff for the results of the histology and eventually one of the more junior members of the team told her that the ulcer had been benign and that she would have no further problems.

On the day before discharge, however, the consultant ward round took place and she was then told by the consultant that the ulcer had shown some early premalignant changes and that she would need regular follow-up, with outpatient consultations and endoscopies in the future. Tania asked the consultant what her prognosis was and the consultant replied that this would depend on a series of regular follow-ups and that the prognosis was uncertain at present. The patient was then discharged home with a follow-up out-patient appointment and a leaflet explaining possible post-gastrectomy symptoms.

Q1 Some elements of this woman's care were suboptimal because of poor communication. Try to list as many of these as you can.

Q2 How could these problems have been avoided?

Clinical case 2 answers

Q1 Failure to exchange information.
  ▪ The patient was not asked about her family history.
  ▪ The patient did not volunteer an important fact in her family history.
  ▪ Her fears about having cancer were not known.
  ▪ Two different versions of her diagnosis were given to her.
  ▪ She was not given clear information about the expected course of her illness and possible prognosis.

Q2 It is advisable that one person should act as a channel for communication where possible, but this is often difficult in the hospital environment where teams of doctors work under the leadership of a consultant and where there is a culture of specialization and referral.

It Tania had been asked by way of an open-ended question about any worries she had prior to the surgery, she might have volunteered the information about her father's death. If the surgical team had been aware of this, the importance of the histology result to her would have been appreciated and an appropriate member of the team could have discussed this with her earlier and answered her questions.

Patients should be made aware that it is reasonable to have several possible management plans and discussions about these different options may take place at the bedside as a teaching tool.

Information should be exchanged with the patient. It is a good idea to give written as well as verbal information to patients.

The patient's GP should be involved whenever possible as he or she can provide continuing support and may be better acquainted with the family circumstances.

Summary

In this Unit, you have studied why the doctor–patient relationship is unbalanced and why this is important. We have discussed the concept of emotional intelligence and why this is especially important when we are dealing with patients. Skills have been identified which are know to be important in developing good communication and building a strong doctor–patient relationship. You should appreciate the importance of attentiveness and the need for active listening techniques in consulations, and understand why empathy is

The doctor–patient relationship

Clinical Topics

C ☐
S ☐
R ☐

important to doctors and patients. Finally, we have emphasized the importance of a patient-centred partnership—and what this actually means!

Surgeons and the law

Author

J. W. R. Peyton

Introduction

This Unit will look in some depth at the rules that govern the practice of medicine. These rules can be defined by custom, by ethical or moral principles, or be enshrined in law. They form the framework that governs our actions and, if infringed, result in varying sanctions from the courts, the General Medical Council (GMC), colleagues or society.

STEP™ Foundation user guide

Work steadily and identify topics that require more work—use a highlighter if you wish, and scribble notes and comments in the wide margins provided. Add links to other useful resources you discover. This will all help you to revise later.

For efficient study, use the tick boxes at the end of each section, writing a date alongside. This will remind you when you have:

- **C** Completed your reading
- **S** Self-assessed using *e*STEP™ Foundation website
- **R** Revised

Do remember to log in to *e*STEP™ Foundation regularly. *e*STEP™ Foundation contains a rich variety of supporting material to make your study more efficient. *e*STEP™ Foundation is updated frequently and will contain late-breaking amendments, unit by unit, as well as valuable additional resources.

 Surgery journal

 eSTEP™ resource

 Textbook

 Weblink

We hope you enjoy working through this Unit. Please use *e*STEP™ Foundation website to provide us with feedback and any comments or suggestions.

Expected learning outcomes

When you have completed this Unit, you will be able to:

- weigh up the ethical, medical and legal principles under which you are permitted to practice medicine
- underpin your duties as a doctor with rulings from seminal local cases
- apply these principles to your every day practice
- recognize the concept of clinical freedom within boundaries regulated by the law, the profession and society in general.

Clinical topics

Clinical topics

Background

Why are rules necessary?

There are three fundamental reasons why societies develop rules to govern behaviour. The first is to develop social cohesion which allows a group to work together with identifiable common aims. A profession which has and acts on a common body of knowledge develops its own internal rules governing members' behaviour, which form the basis of ethics. Secondly, rules are required to maintain order in society and to define 'right' and 'wrong' behaviour. Individuals with different views are coerced into acceptable behaviour for the common good. Finally, recognition of the rights of individuals to develop, means that the rule of law may have to be used to balance competing interests between individuals or between an individual and society.

What is the basis of the rules?

The first is custom. In the medical world this relates to the expectations of patients who are asked to put their trust in doctors and nurses. Simple examples are the white coat or a nurse's uniform, which give the impression of authority, stability and dependability.

The second basis are ethical and moral principles, which differ from those enshrined in law, although over time the two tend to merge. Attitudes towards abortion illustrate a moral issue not enshrined in law. Different groups in society, and indeed within the medical profession, have differing views on the morality of abortion. However, in certain circumstances, abortion is legal and patients have the right to be referred to another practitioner if their own GP disapproves: similarly with contraceptive advice. A very common ethical issue involves relationships with patients. There exist no moral or legal bars to liaisons between unmarried persons. However, a close social relationship between a doctor and patient is not acceptable from an ethical point of view. Finally, an ambulance speeding to an emergency is breaking the law if it exceeds the speed limit. Morally it may be regarded as appropriate in order to save life, but being in a hurry is not a defence if an accident ensues.

The law and medicine

We will consider a number of cases which have been fundamental in shaping the law as it stands today. Most deal with medical issues but others do not. The reason they are important is the principle of *stare decisis* (Latin 'to stand by that which is decided') by which courts apply precedent to cases involving similar facts. A brief summary of the facts of each case is set out in the unit. You are then asked to decide the relevant issues and how they influence medical practice. You are then given excerpts from the judgement to consider, and finally feedback on how the outcome of each case has influenced clinicians. By the end of this unit, you should have a clear understanding of the legal background to some of the decisions you will have to make in everyday practice, understanding that the legal position is constantly evolving, as does society itself.

Duty of care

Barnett v The Chelsea and Kensington Hospital Management Committee
[1969] 1 QBD 428

Facts

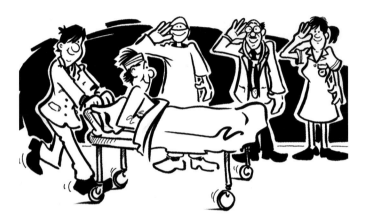

Three night watchmen arrived at a hospital casualty department, having been driven there by William Patrick Barnett, who eventually died. There was no one on duty at the reception desk, and they met the nurse on duty in the middle of the casualty department. They complained that they had been vomiting continuously for 3 hours after drinking tea and asked to see a doctor. Mr Barnett did not actually speak to the nurse, but lay down on some chairs.

The nurse's first impression was that the men had been drinking excessively. One became angry and demanded to see a doctor. The nurse telephoned the casualty officer on duty and told him that the three men had been vomiting after drinking tea. The doctor replied, 'Well, I am vomiting myself and I have not been drinking. Tell them to go home and go to bed and call their own doctors.'

The men left and approximately 5 hours later Mr Barnett died. It turned out that this was due to poisoning by arsenic that had contaminated the tea.

Learning exercise	1

What are the main issues of this case?

Answer to learning exercise

1   The issues are:

    a When patients arrive at a casualty department, can they demand treatment from a doctor?

    b Did the casualty officer fail in his duty by not examining the patients?

    c What is the legal definition of negligence and does it apply in this case?

▼

Excerpts from the judgement of Justice Nield

I turn to consider the nature of the duty which the law imposes on persons in the position of the defendants and their servants and agents. The problem ... is to determine the duty of those who provide and run a casualty department when a person presents themselves at that department complaining of illness or injury and before he has been treated and received into the hospital wards.

This is not a case of a casualty department which closes its doors and says that no patients can be received. Three watchmen entered the defendant's hospital without hindrance, they made complaints to the nurse who received them and she in turn passed those complaints to the casualty officer and he sent a message through the nurse purporting to advise the three men.

Thus I have no doubt that Nurse Corbett and the medical casualty officer were under a duty to the deceased to exercise that skill and care which is to be expected of persons in such positions acting reasonably.

It is not, in my judgement, the case that a casualty officer must always see the caller at his department. Casualty departments are misused from time to time [for instance] ... if the caller has a small cut which the nurse can perfectly well dress herself, then the casualty officer need not be called. However without a doubt the casualty officer should have seen and examined the deceased. His failure to do either cannot be described as an excusable error as has been submitted. It was negligence. It is unfortunate he was himself at the time a tired and unwell doctor, but there was no one else to do that which was his duty to do.

Comment

In this case, the doctor had a duty to see the watchmen and, in failing to do so, breached this duty. However, in legal terms, in order to substantiate a claim for negligence, some form of damage must result to the plaintiff because of the breach: the classic triad of duty, breach and damage.

Here, however, the judge decided that it was unlikely that any treatment that could have been started by the time Mr Barnett would have been admitted to the ward (for example, the use of British Anti-Lewisite or BAL—an antidote to an obsolete arsenic based chemical warfare agent) could have prevented his death. Therefore, the claim for negligence actually failed.

Learning exercise	2

What does this mean for your clinical practice?

Answer to learning exercise

2   If a casualty department is open, the staff working in it have a duty to see any patient who turns up. Except in the most minor cases, the casualty officer has a duty to see and examine all patients and in general terms advice over the phone is not acceptable.

This case also introduces the legal definition which allows a claim for negligence to arise against a doctor: there must exist a duty of care, it must be breached and damage must occur as a consequence of the breach.

In the case of a doctor, this obviously arises in the workplace but, under English law, does not extend to social activities, for example at a party or in an aircraft. However, once a doctor accepts responsibility for a patient, he or she then has a continuing duty to look after them or hand them over to another competent practitioner. Breach of this duty becomes actionable in court if any damage occurs as a direct result of the breach. This does not mean that a doctor cannot be held responsible for a breach of duty where no damage occurs, but these cases would fall more into the realm of a disciplinary action by the employer or, in more serious cases, by the GMC.

The duties and standards of a doctor registered with the GMC are stipulated in the publication *Good Medical Practice (Protecting Patients, Guiding Doctors)*. You may obtain an up to date copy of this document via *e*STEP™ Foundation. You should now study the booklet carefully as it clearly lays down the standards against which you will be judged in terms of your professional practice.

Standard of care

Incompetence

An incompetent practitioner is one who falls below recognized standards of care. Remember, a standard of care is, by definition, the lowest acceptable level of performance and does not equate to best medical practice, to which all practitioners should aspire.

Quality of care

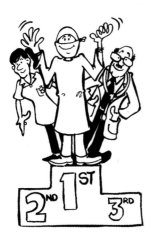

Wells v Cooper [1958] 2 QBD 265

Facts

Mr Wells was a fishmonger and had delivered fish at the house of Mr Cooper. When leaving, he pulled the door and the handle came off in his hand. He fell 4 feet from a platform and was injured.

C ☐
S ☐
R ☐

The handle had been attached to the door 4 or 5 months previously by Mr Cooper who used three-quarter inch screws. He was well accustomed to doing small repair jobs about the house and he believed that the handle was perfectly secure. In this instance, his method of fixation proved inadequate.

Learning exercise 3

What are the main issues of this case?

Answer to learning exercise

3 The issues are:

a Could Mr Cooper have foreseen that if the handle came away when a person pulled the door shut, that the person might suffer injury?

b Ought Mr Cooper to have known that the screws were not adequate?

Excerpts from the judgement of Lord Justice Jenkins

Accordingly, we think that the defendant did nothing unreasonable in undertaking the work himself. But it behoved him, if he was to discharge his duty of care to persons such as the plaintiff, to do work with reasonable care and skill and we think there is a degree of care and skill required of him which must be measured, not by reference to the degree of competence in such matters which he personally happened to possess, but by reference to the degree of care and skill which a reasonably competent carpenter might be expected to apply to the work in question.

It cannot be that the standard of care to be required of someone who does the relevant work himself is lower than it would have been if he had employed an independent contractor to do it for him.

Comment

This case is highly relevant to the standard of care required towards other people and, in particular, patients. Note Lord Denning's discussion of standard of care in the next case.

Nettleship v Weston [1971] 2 QBD 691

Facts

Mrs Weston wanted to learn to drive. She asked a friend, Mr Nettleship, if he could give her some lessons. He agreed to do so providing he was fully insured.

On her third lesson she pulled out of a junction, turned the steering wheel to the left and the car moved around the corner at a walking pace. Mr Nettleship told her to straighten up but she did not do so. She panicked and held the wheel tightly. Mr Nettleship tried to straighten the car up but it mounted the kerb and struck a lamp post. Mr Nettleship was injured, fracturing his left patella.

Learning exercise 4

What are the main issues of this case?

Answer to learning exercise

4   The issues are:

    a What is the duty of care owed by a learner driver under instruction to passengers or the public at large?

    b What is the duty of care of the instructor?

Excerpts from the judgement of Lord Denning, Master of the Rolls, and Lord Justice Megaw

Per *Lord Denning*

In civil law, if a driver goes off the road onto a pavement and injures a pedestrian, or damages property, he is *prima facie* (Latin for 'at first view' or 'on its face') liable. It is not an answer for him to say, 'I was a learner driver under instruction. I was doing my best but could not help it.' The civil law permits no such excuse. It requires of him the same standard of care as any other driver. The learner driver may be doing his best, but his incompetent best is not good enough. He must drive in as good a manner as a driver of skill, experience and care who is sound in mind and limb, who makes no errors of judgement, has good eyesight and hearing and is free from any infirmity.

I regard the learner driver and the instructor as both concerned in the driving. Together they must maintain the same measure of control over the car as an experienced, skilled and careful driver would do. That is, I think, obvious. Their joint driving must come up to the high standard required of a single individual. If there is an accident, such as would not have occurred with a careful driver, then one or other, or both, must have been at fault.

Per *Lord Justice Megaw*

Why should the doctrine, if it be part of the law, be limited to cases involved in the driving of motor cars? Suppose that to the knowledge of the patient a young surgeon, whom the patient has chosen to operate on him, has only just qualified. If the operation goes wrong because of the surgeon's inexperience, is there a defence on the basis that the standard of skill and care is lower than the standard of a common and experienced surgeon?

Learning exercise   5

What does this mean for your clinical practice?

Answer to learning exercise

5   Here Justice Megaw was discussing a newly qualified consultant. These cases give an indication of the court's view of the standards of care required of a junior doctor in training or even a senior doctor learning a operation.

You will note that it is not acceptable to make a mistake 'just because you are a learner'. If you operate on anyone, you are expected to carry out the procedure with the skill of a competent practitioner and nothing less is acceptable. Further, it is quite clear that anyone who is with you at the operating table has joint responsibility for anything that happens. This therefore applies to you whether you are under instruction, or helping someone with less experience through an operative procedure.

C ☐
S ☐
R ☐

These cases have therefore warned you not to undertake procedures in which you have not been fully trained without a more experienced colleague. Further, you must not allow anyone under your direction to undertake procedures in which they are not fully trained, since you will be jointly liable for any problems that arise, whether or not you are present. Note that this applies not only in the operating room, but also in the ward or out-patients department. Beware of giving or receiving advice over the telephone.

The consultant in charge of the case has overall responsibility whether or not he is actually present at the operating table. It is important not only that you feel competent to undertake a procedure, but also that the consultant has a similar confidence in your abilities. These issues should be clarified in advance of undertaking any procedure whether elective or emergency. It has to be accepted that even in a case that appears to be routine, surprises can occur and you may not be competent to deal with the new situation. Therefore, it is vital that at all times you have means of communicating with your consultant so that he or she may give advice or attend directly if necessary.

Level of knowledge

Roe (and Woolley) v Ministry of Health and others [1954] 2 All ER 131

Facts

On 13 October 1947 both plaintiffs underwent a surgical operation under spinal anaesthetic. This consisted of nupercaine, injected by means of a lumbar puncture, and was administered to the patients by the second defendant, who was a specialist anaesthetist. The nupercaine was contained in glass ampoules which were, prior to use, immersed in a phenol solution. After the operations, both plaintiffs developed spastic paraplegia which resulted in permanent paralysis from the waist downwards.

The ampoules were supplied in a box. There was a notice on the box which stated that they were to be treated as 'frankly septic' as they were not sterilized. The practice at that time was to place them into phenol. However, it transpired on this occasion that the phenol had percolated into the nupercaine through molecular flaws or invisible cracks in the ampoules. At the time of the operations, this risk was appreciated if there were obvious cracks in the glass, but contamination was not expected to occur at the molecular level.

Learning exercise	6

What is the main issue of this case?

Answer to learning exercise

6 The main issue is 'what was the level of knowledge of a competent anaesthetist on the date in question?'

Excerpts from the judgement of Lord Justice Denning

The crack was of a kind that no one in any experiment has been able to reproduce again. It was too blind to be seen, but it was enough to let in sufficient phenol to corrode the nerves, whilst still leaving enough nupercaine to anaesthetize the patient. And this very exceptional crack occurred, not in one ampoule only, but in two ampoules used on the same day in two successive operations; and none of the other ampoules was damaged at all.

This has taught the doctors to be on their guard against invisible cracks. Never again, it is to be hoped, would such a thing happen. After this accident a leading text book by Professor Mackintosh on Lumbar Puncture and Spinal Anaesthesia, was published in 1951 which contains the significant warning:

Never place ampoules of local anaesthetic solution in alcohol or spirits. This common practice is probably responsible for some of the cases of permanent paralysis reported after spinal analgesia.

If the hospitals were to continue the practice after this warning, they could not complain if they were found guilty of negligence. But the warning had not been given at the time of this accident. Indeed, it was the extraordinary accident of these two men which first disclosed the danger. Nowadays it would be negligent not to realize the danger, but it was not then.

One final word. These two men have suffered such terrible consequences that there is a natural feeling they should be compensated. But we should be doing a disservice to the community at large if we were to impose liability on hospitals and doctors for everything that happens to go wrong. Doctors would be led to think more of their own safety than the good of their patients. Initiative would be stifled and confidence shaken. A proper sense of proportion requires us to have regard to the conditions in which hospitals and doctors have to work. We must insist on due care for the patient at every point, but we must not condemn as negligence that which is only a misadventure.

Learning exercise	7

What does this mean for your clinical practice?

Answer to learning exercise

7   This case clearly demonstrates that the standard of care you are required to provide

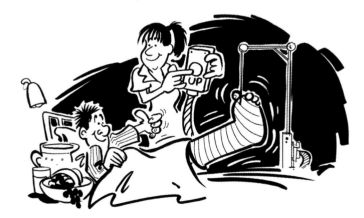

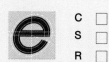

C ☐
S ☐
R ☐

for your patients is that level which is expected of you at the date you are actually providing the treatment. All of us will be involved in cases which may take many years to come to court and, indeed, may be asked in the future to comment on the care that others provided a number of years ago. We must be careful to explore the body of medical opinion at the time the incident occurred and the conditions which pertained at the time.

Further, there is a clear warning about keeping up to date with medical and technical literature, especially on safety issues involving drugs or equipment. A lack of knowledge about recent issues is not acceptable, which makes it very difficult to stray outside your field of expertise into other areas about which you may have occasional knowledge from your past experience.

It is also of interest that Lord Denning foresaw the onset of 'defensive medicine'. As a doctor you must not be afraid to move forwards and to innovate, but you must have very good reasons to depart from normal practice. Evidence-based medicine should not be seen to stifle progress, but rather to make that progress more logical and scientific, not just in your mind but also to the profession and the public at large.

Confidentiality

Attorney General v Mulholland & Foster [1963] 1 All ER 266 (*v Foster*)

Facts

A tribunal was set up to look into circumstances in which alleged offences under the Official Secrets Act were committed by Vassal. In particular, allegations reflecting on the honour and integrity of persons who, as ministers, naval officers or civil servants, neglected their duty in allowing Vassal's employment on secret work for the government.

Mulholland had written articles for a newspaper that Vassal was known in the Admiralty as 'Auntie' to his face, that a female typist had decided that no £15 per week clerk could possibly live the way he did honestly, and that it was the sponsorship of Vassal by two high-ranking officials which allowed Vassal to avoid the strictest part of the Admiralty's security vetting.

Foster wrote an article for his newspaper and in one passage asked why the spy-catchers failed to notice Vassal, who sometimes wore women's clothing on West End trips. Both Mulholland and Foster were asked to disclose the sources of their information and refused.

Learning exercise	8

What are the main issues of this case?

Answer to learning exercise

8   The issues are:

a   What is the nature of confidentiality?

b   Under what circumstances does information given in confidence have to be divulged?

Excerpts from the judgement of Lord Denning, Master of the Rolls

It appears that allegations were made in some newspapers which reflected gravely on persons in high places and on naval officers and civil servants in the Admiralty. The articles clearly imported that there had been neglect of duty on their part, in not discovering a spy was in their midst.

In the course of the enquiry, the journalists responsible for these articles were asked to give their sources of information and they refused to answer. Was this a question which they could legally be required to answer? That depends on two questions: First, was it relevant and necessary in this sense, that it was a question that ought to be answered to enable proper investigation to be made? Second, if it was, have the journalists a privilege in point of law to refuse an answer? Under the statute, any witness before a tribunal is entitled to the same immunities and privileges as if he were a witness before the High Court.

Then it is said that, however relevant these questions were and however proper to be answered or the purpose of the enquiry, a journalist has a privilege by law entitling him to refuse to give his sources of information. The journalist puts forward his justification as the pursuit of truth.

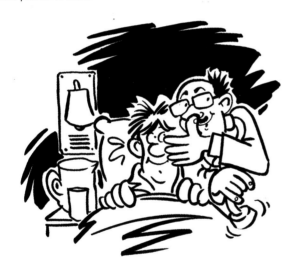

The only profession that I know which is given a privilege from disclosing information to a court of law is the legal profession, and then it is not the privilege of the lawyer but of his client. Take a clergyman, the banker or the medical man, none of these is entitled to refuse to answer when directed by a judge. Let me not be mistaken. The judge will respect the confidence which each member of these honourable professions receives in the course of it, and will not direct him to answer unless not only is it relevant but also a proper and, indeed, necessary question in the course of justice to be put and answered. A judge is the person entrusted, on behalf of the community, to weigh these conflicting interests. If the judge determines the journalist must answer, then no privilege will avail him to refuse.

What does this mean for your clinical practice?

Answer to learning exercise

9 This case is very important in the matter of confidentiality. Indeed, Lord Justice Donovan in the same case stated this would apply not only in the case of journalists but also in other cases where information is given and received under the seal of confidence, for example, information given by a patient to their doctor arising out of that relationship. In other words, the privilege of confidentiality is not absolute. A judge always has the utmost discretion as to whether or not the information must be disclosed. However, patients do have a right to expect that under normal circumstances information given to you in confidence should not be disclosed unless they give permission. You are therefore under a duty to make sure that information given to you is reasonably protected and not disclosed to anyone else unless there are exceptional circumstances.

The GMC has produced a booklet entitled *Confidentiality*, which you should now take time to read. You may download the latest version via an *e*STEP™ Foundation link. You will undoubtedly be asked many times in your career about information in relation to your patients, for example by relatives, for research purposes or by the police. You therefore must have a clear understanding of the circumstances under which it is acceptable for you to discuss your patient with a third party.

Clinical case 1

Mrs Wilson is 68 years old and has just been diagnosed by you as having breast cancer with metastases in her liver, spine and left lung.

Q1 How might it be argued that to inform the relatives before informing Mrs Wilson of the terminal nature of her illness, would be a violation of her moral right to confidentiality?

Q2 Under what circumstances are breaches of confidentiality legally required by surgeons?

Q3 Under what circumstances are breaches of confidentiality discretionary for surgeons?

Clinical case 1 answers

Q1 Mrs Wilson is a competent adult whose autonomy should be respected. Just as she has a moral right to provide informed consent to surgical treatment, she should be able to exercise control over clinical information about herself. She might not want her relatives to hear about the seriousness of her condition from anyone but herself. Indeed, she may not want them to know at all. Equally, her relatives may wish her ill. For example, they may know that she has been thinking of changing her will to their disadvantage and believe that she will certainly do so if she realizes how ill she is.

Surgeons should remember that they cannot necessarily assume that relationships within families are always as good as they appear to be on the surface. A breach of confidence may lead to harm to the patient and, if discovered, to a loss of trust in the surgeon.

Q2 Breaches of confidence are mandatory under the following circumstances:

⊓ When a judge demands it—either through an order issued by the court to give up clinical records or by the judge in court after the issue of a subpoena.

⊓ In the case of notifiable diseases.

⊓ For use as evidence in an NHS tribunal.

⊓ When a patient is suspected of terrorism within the UK.

Q3 Breaches of confidence are discretionary:

⊓ When the surgeon has evidence that a patient may pose a serious risk to others through criminal activities.

⊓ When there is other evidence of such a threat, for example a patient suffering from epilepsy who will not report to the Licensing Authority.

⊓ When respecting confidentiality would place a named individual at risk of death or serious harm.

When considering such breaches, surgeons should always remember that they are accountable and may be asked to justify their actions. Patients should be informed when a breach of confidence is considered.

Negligence

Bolithio v City and Hackney Health Authority [1997] 4 All ER 771

Facts

On 16 January 1994, a 12-year-old boy was admitted to hospital with a diagnosis of croup and a respiratory wheeze. He was examined by the paediatric senior house officer who arranged for him to have some special nursing overnight. The following morning he appeared to be much better and was seen by the consultant. His clinical condition was improving and he ate a large lunch.

At 12.40 pm he was having great difficulty breathing and the ward sister contacted the senior paediatric registrar because she was very concerned about his condition. The doctor stated she would be there as soon as possible but, in the event, did not come. The child seemed to recover spontaneously. However, at 2.00 pm he again had considerable difficulty in breathing. The ward sister told the senior registrar, who told her to ask the senior house officer to see the child. Neither doctor responded to the call. He seemed to recover again, but at 2.30 pm he became agitated and began to cry. Whilst the nurse was phoning the doctors the child collapsed. He suffered a cardiac arrest. He was revived after 9–10 minutes but sustained severe brain damage from which he subsequently died.

Learning exercise   10

What are the main issues of this case?

Answer to learning exercise

10 The issues are:

a Were the doctors negligent in not attending the child when asked to do so by the ward sister?

b What action would the doctors have undertaken if they had attended and would it have made any difference to the eventual outcome?

c Most importantly, if they did follow a course of action such as would be approved by a group of senior doctors, would that protect them from a claim for negligence if another group of senior doctors fundamentally disagreed with their management?

Excerpts from the judgement of Lord Browne-Wilkinson

The defendants accepted that the senior paediatric registrar was in breach of her duty of care after receiving telephone calls not to have attended a child or arranged for a suitable deputy to do so.

Negligence having been established, the question had to be decided, would the cardiac arrest have been avoided if the senior registrar or some other suitable deputy had attended as they should have done. By the end of the trial it was common ground, first, that intubation so as to provide an airway in any event would have ensured that the respiratory failure which occurred did not lead to cardiac arrest and, second, that such intubation would have had to be carried out, if at all, before the final catastrophic episode.

[It was accepted that] had the senior registrar come to see the child at 2.00 pm, she would not have arranged for him to be intubated. However, the judge found that she would have made preparation to ensure that a speedy intubation could take place. In the event that proved to be an irrelevant finding since the judge found that such preparation would have made no difference to the outcome.

The original trial judge had evidence from no less than eight medical experts, all of them distinguished. Five of them were called on behalf of the child and all were of the view that, at least after the second episode, any competent doctor would have intubated. On the other side, the defendants called three experts, all of whom said that, on the symptoms presented by the child as recounted by the sister and the nurse, intubation would not have been appropriate.

The trial judge held that the views of the experts, though diametrically opposed, both represented a responsible body of professional opinion espoused by distinguished and truthful experts. Therefore, he held that Doctor Horn, if she had attended and not intubated, would have come up to a proper level of skill and competence.

My Lord, I agree with these submissions to the extent that, in my view, the court is not bound to hold that a defendant doctor escapes liability for negligence, treatment or diagnosis just because he leads evidence from a number of medical experts who are genuinely of the opinion that the defendant's treatment or diagnosis accorded with sound medical practice.

In *Bolam's* case [1957] 2 All ER 118, McNair J stated that the defendant had to have acted in accordance with the practice accepted as proper by a responsible body of medical men. Later he referred to a standard of practice recognized as proper by a competent reasonable body of opinion. The use of these adjectives — responsible, reasonable and respectable — all show that the court has to be satisfied that the exponents of a body of opinion relied on can demonstrate that such opinion has a logical basis. In particular, in cases involving, as they so often do, the weighing of risks against benefits, the judge before accepting a body of opinion as being responsible, reasonable or respectable, would need to be satisfied that, in forming their views, the experts have directed their minds to the question of comparative risks and benefits and have reached a defensible conclusion in the matter.

Learning exercise	11

What does this mean for your clinical practice?

Answer to learning exercise

11   The *Bolam* case referred to in Browne-Wilkinson's judgement was settled in 1957. Before the *Bolithio* case, it was assumed that the law meant if a doctor was accused of negligently treating a patient, all he or she had to do was find a number of other doctors who would have managed the patient's treatment in the same manner and the court would have to accept that the doctor's treatment was reasonable. This has now been qualified by *Bolithio* in that there must be a clear, logical reason for the method of treatment. As McNair stated in a later part of his judgement, 'a doctor is not negligent, if he has acted in accordance with such a practice, merely because there is a body of opinion which takes a contrary view. At the same time, that does not mean that a medical man can obstinately and pig-headedly carry on with some old technique if it has been proved to be contrary to what is really substantially the whole of informed medical opinion. Otherwise you might get men today saying "I don't believe in anaesthetics and I don't believe in antiseptics, I am going to continue to do my surgery in the way it was done in the 18th century".' That clearly would be wrong.

This judgement is at the heart of the issues of clinical governance, which has been defined as corporate responsibility for clinical practice. This is basically a quality issue and it is a means whereby Trust management can ensure that staff are adequately trained and are continually updated. There is a need for a system whereby good practice and evidence-based innovations can be systemically disseminated and implemented.

When you finish your training, you will have a body of knowledge and be recognized by your peers as being a competent, capable practitioner. However, the practice of medicine changes very quickly and doctors are required to be involved in life-long learning, a process known as continuing professional development (CPD). You must be able critically to review all the information you are given about changes in your practice whether from colleagues, conferences or journals. You must decide whether there is a sound reason for you to change your practice and must be prepared

C ☐
S ☐
R ☐

logically to defend your decisions if they are challenged. This is the underlying concept of evidence-based medicine.

In lay terms, negligence is an ethical issue relating to those who breach their duty of care. The legal definition of negligence goes further and requires that some damage must have occurred to the patient as a result of the breach of duty. Therefore, a doctor can be ethically negligent and answerable to the GMC but not be open to a civil claim of negligence because no damage ensued from the breach of care. Legal negligence requires the classic triad of duty, breach and damage.

Gross negligence

R v Adomako [1994] 5 Med LR 27

Facts

Dr Adomako was the anaesthetist during an eye operation. He did not notice that the ventilator had become disconnected for 6 minutes. As a result, the patient suffered a cardiac arrest and died. He was charged with manslaughter.

Learning exercise	12

What are the issues of this case?

Answer to learning exercise

12 The issues are:

  a Was he negligent?

  b Was that negligence sufficient to result in a criminal action?

Excerpts from the judgement

There was no dispute that Dr Adomako had been negligent. He had a clear duty, it was breached, as a result of which the patient died. The legal triad of duty, breach and damage therefore was easily proved.

Per *The Lord Chancellor*

The essence of the matter, which is supremely a jury question, is whether, having regard to the risk of death involved, the conduct of the defendant was so bad in all circumstances as to amount in their judgement to a criminal act or omission. Therefore, in order to secure a conviction for manslaughter, the conduct of the defendant causing death must:

1 have fallen far below the standard to be expected of a reasonable doctor (in this case a competent anaesthetist);

2 have involved a risk of death; and

3 have been so bad that all the circumstances, as in the opinion of the jury, amount to a crime.

So we must conclude there is a head [category] of manslaughter which at least includes causing death by an act done, being aware it is highly probable that it will cause serious bodily harm.

Learning exercise   13

What does this mean for your clinical practice?

Answer to learning exercise

13 Paradoxically, this case actually offers greater protection to doctors in their clinical practice, since prior to it, it was relatively easy for them to be caught by a concept of recklessness and therefore charged with manslaughter.

Gross negligence has to be much more than just reckless behaviour but behaviour that is reckless to such an extent as to be worthy of criminal sanction. Nonetheless, if doctors either perform an act or omit to perform an act and should be aware that because of this action it is highly probable death may occur, they are laying themselves open to a charge of manslaughter at whatever level of training.

C ☐
S ☐
R ☐

Consent

Trespass

Wilson v Pringle [1986] 3 WLR 1

Facts

In December 1980, both parties were schoolboys aged 13. On the day of the incident, both were in a corridor at school and the plaintiff was carrying a school bag over his right shoulder. The bag was of the hand grip type and the plaintiff was holding the handle in his right hand and holding the bag over his shoulders so that the bag hung down his back. The defendant pulled the bag off the plaintiff's shoulder and the plaintiff fell hurting his hip. The defendant claimed that it was an act of ordinary horseplay between pupils in the same school and the damage was not intentional.

Learning exercise   14

What is the main issue of this case?

Answer to learning exercise

14 The issue is the unintentional touching of another person which results in damage is negligence. The intentional touching of another person constitutes trespass. There are only a few defences to trespass, one of which is consent.

Excerpts from the judgement of Lord Justice Croom-Johnston

Defences to an action for trespass to the person, such as consent, provide a solution to the old problem of what legal rule allows a surgeon to perform an operation on an unconscious patient who is brought into hospital. The patient cannot consent, and there may be no next of kin available to do it for him. Hitherto it has been customary to say that in such cases, consent is to be implied for what would otherwise be a battery on the unconscious body. It is better simply to say that the surgeon's action is acceptable in ordinary conduct of everyday life and not a battery.

Comment

Does this mean that consent necessarily allows a surgeon to perform whatever action he or she wishes? The next case considers this further.

R v Brown and other appeals [1993] 2 All ER 75

Facts

The appellants belonged to a group of sado-masochistic homosexuals who, over a long period of time, participated in the commission of acts of violence against each other for sexual pleasure. The passive partner in each case consented to the acts being committed and suffered no permanent injury. The activities took place in private; video cameras were used to record the activities, but the tapes were not sold or used other than for the delectation of members of the group.

Learning exercise	15

What is the main issue of this case?

Answer to learning exercise

15   The issue is whether or not an adult can legally consent to being wounded by another.

Excerpts from the judgement of Lord Templeman

In some circumstances, violence is not punishable under the criminal law. When no actual bodily harm was caused, the consenting person affected is precluded from complaining. There can be no conviction for the summary offence of common assault if the victim has consented to the assault. Even when the violence is intentionally inflicted and results in actual bodily harm, wounding or serious bodily harm, the accused is entitled to be acquitted if the injury was a foreseeable incident arising out of a lawful activity in which the person injured was participating.

Surgery involves intentional violence resulting in actual or sometimes serious bodily harm, but surgery is a lawful activity. Other activities carried on with consent by or on behalf of the injured person have been accepted as lawful notwithstanding that they involve actual bodily harm or may cause some serious bodily harm. Ritual circumcision, tattooing, ear piercing and sports including boxing are lawful activities.

Per *Lord Mustill*

Many of the acts done by surgeons would be very serious crimes if done by anyone else and yet surgeons incur no liability. Actual consent, or the substitute for consent deemed by law to exist where an emergency creates a need for action, is the essential element in this immunity; but it cannot be a direct explanation for it since much of the bodily invasion involved in surgery lies well above the point which consent could even arguably be regarded as furnishing a defence. Why is it so? The answer must, in my opinion, be proper medical treatment, for which actual or seemed consent is a prerequisite, in a category in its own.

Learning exercise   16

What do these cases mean for your clinical practice?

Answer to learning exercise

16   Surgeons are placed in a very special position as regards their patients. This is a relationship of trust—or a fiduciary relationship. Surgery is lawful providing there is consent, unless in an emergency situation, when the doctor has a duty to do what is best for the patient. Consent must be informed and the doctor has no right to inflict injury against the expressed wishes of a patient. This includes not only surgical intervention, but also activities such as taking blood or inserting a drip.

Further, certain operations which are not done for the benefit of the patient can also be called into question. It is of note that in the judgement above, ritual circumcision is mentioned. If this is not carried out for the benefit of the patient then it is unlawful. Particular mention has been made in the recent past of female circumcision and the big outcry when it was realized that some operations were being performed by surgeons in England at the request of families.

You must be quite clear that you are not entitled to perform any procedure unless it arises from a duty of care to patients and is for their benefit. These considerations must be uppermost in a practitioner's mind at all times and perhaps particularly when discussing new methods of treatment, whether these are of a surgical nature or, for instance, research into the action of new drugs. If the practitioner cannot convince a judge that the treatment was for the benefit of the patient, then they lay themselves open to a charge of assault.

Informed consent

C ☐
S ☐
R ☐

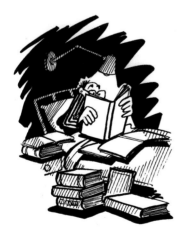

Sidaway v Board of Governors of Bethlem Royal Hospital and Maudsley Hospital [1985] 1 AC 871

Facts

Mrs Sidaway suffered severe pain in her neck, right shoulder and arms. This was due to a deformity of the fifth and sixth cervical vertebrae. Conservation treatment including a collar, traction and manipulation did not cure the matter, nor did a fusion carried out in 1960.

In 1973 she was again suffering from increased pain and this was diagnosed as being the result of pressure on the fourth cervical nerve root. In October 1974 she underwent surgery, which consisted of a laminectomy on the fourth cervical vertebra and a foraminectomy of disc space between the fourth and fifth cervical vertebrae. At operation, the fourth cervical nerve root was freed by removing the facets from the fourth vertebra using a dental drill. Post-operatively Mrs Sidaway was recorded as being severely disabled by a partial paralysis resulting from the operation. She stated that had she known the possibility of such an outcome, she would never have consented to the procedure.

Learning exercise   17

What are the main issues of this case?

Answer to learning exercise

17   The issues are:

  a   What is the basis of the claim of negligence against the surgeon and his employers?

  b   How much information is required by a 'prudent patient' in order to decide whether or not they will consent to an operation?

Excerpts from the judgements

By the time this case came to appeal, it had been agreed that the surgeon had performed the operation with due care and skill. The issue raised in the judgement was the warning which the surgeon gave his patients of the specific risks inherent in the operation. All the surgeons called as expert witnesses accepted that the risk of damage, though slight, was a real one. They distinguished between two categories of specific risk: the effect of damage to a nerve root, being in all probability that the operation would fail to relieve and might increase pain; and damage to the spinal cord, which might cause partial paralysis. The risk of damage to the spinal cord was, however, in their opinion less than 1% and the risk of damage to the nerve between 1% and 2%.

Per *Lord Scarman*

The *Bolam* principle may be formulated as a rule that a doctor is not negligent if he acts in accordance with the practice accepted at the time as proper by a responsible body of medical opinion even though other doctors adopt a different practice. In short, the law imposes the duty of care, but the standard of care is a matter of medical judgement.

The implications of this view of the law are disturbing. It leaves the determination of legal duty to the judgement of doctors. Responsible medical judgement may, indeed, provide law with an acceptable standard in determining whether a doctor in diagnosis or treatment had complied with his duty. But is it right that medical judgement should determine whether there exists a duty to warn of risk and its scope? It would be a strange conclusion if the courts should be led to conclude that our law, which undoubtedly recognizes a right in the patient to decide whether he would accept or reject the treatment proposed, should permit the doctors to determine whether and in what circumstances a duty arises requiring the doctor to warn his patient of the risk inherent in the treatment which he proposes.

A doctor who operates without the consent of a patient is, save in cases of emergency or mental disability, guilty of the civil wrong of trespass to the person. He is also guilty of a criminal offence of assault.

The existence of a patient's right to make his own decision, which may be seen as a basic human right protected by the common law, is a reason why a doctrine embodying a right of the patient to be informed of the risks of surgical treatment has been developed in some jurisdictions in the USA and has found favour in the Supreme Court of Canada. Known as the doctrine of informed consent, it amounts to this.

Where there is a real or material risk inherent in the proposed operation (however competently and skilfully performed), the question whether and to what extent the patient should be warned before he gives his consent is to be answered not by reference to medical practice but by accepting as a matter of law, subject to all proper exceptions (of which the Court, not the profession, is the judge), a patient has a right to be informed of the risks inherent in the treatment which is proposed.

In *Canterbury v Spence* (an American case) the court enunciated four propositions:

1 The root premise is the concept that every human being of adult years and of sound mind has the right to determine what shall be done with his own body.

2 The consent is the informed exercise of a choice and that entails an opportunity to evaluate knowledgeably the options available and the risks attendant upon each.

3 The doctrine must therefore disclose all material risks; what risks are material are determined by the prudent patient test which is 'a risk is ... material when a reasonable person, in what the physician knows or should know to be the patient's position, would be likely to attach significance to the risk or cluster of risks in deciding whether or not to forego the proposed therapy'.

4 The doctor, however, has what the court called a therapeutic privilege. This exception enables a doctor to withhold from his patient information as to risk, if it can be shown that a reasonable medical assessment of the patient would have indicated to the doctor that disclosure would have posed a serious threat of psychological detriment.

My conclusion as to the law is therefore this. To the extent that I have indicated, I think that English law must recognize a duty of the doctor to warn his patient of risk and adhere to the treatment which he is proposing, and especially so if the treatment be surgery. The critical limitation is that the duty is confined to material risk. The test of materiality is whether in the circumstances of a particular case, the court is satisfied that a reasonable person in the patient's position would be likely to attach significance to the risk. Even if the risk be material, the doctor will not be liable if upon a reasonable assessment of his patient's condition he takes the view that a warning would be detrimental to his patient's health.

Per *Lord Diplock*

The combined chance [of damage to the nerve or the spinal column] was put at something below 2%, of which injury to the spinal cord was rather more likely to have serious consequence if it were to happen, but the chance of its happening was less than half the chance of damage to the nerve roots, i.e. less than one in a hundred.

Those members of the public who seek medical or surgical advice would be badly served by the adoption of any legal principle which would confine the doctor to some long established, well tried method of treatment only. Although its past record of success might be small, if he wanted to be competent he could not run the risk of being held liable in negligence simply because he tried some more modern treatment, and by some unavoidable mischance had failed to heal but did some harm to the patient. This would encourage defensive medicine with a vengeance.

Per *Lord Bridge*

I am of the opinion that the judge might in certain circumstances come to the conclusion that the disclosure of particular risk was so obviously necessary to an informed choice on the part of a patient that no reasonably prudent medical man would fail to make it. The kind of case I have in mind would be an operation involving substantial risk of grave adverse consequences, as, for example, 10% risk of a stroke. In such a case, in the absence of some cogent clinical reason why a patient should not be informed, a doctor, respecting his patient's right of decision, could hardly fail to appreciate the necessity for appropriate warning.

In the instant case, I can see no reasonable ground on which the judge could properly reject the conclusion to which the unchallenged medical evidence led in the application of the *Bolam* test. The trial judge's assessment of the risk at 1% or 2% covered both nerve root and spinal cord damage and covered a spectrum of possible ill effects ranging from the mild to the catastrophic. In these circumstances, the balance of expert witness agreement that the nondisclosure complained of accorded, with the practice accepted as proper by a responsible body of neurosurgical opinion, afforded the respondents complete defence to the claim.

Per *Lord Templeman*

In my opinion, if a patient knows that a major operation may entail serious consequences, the patient cannot complain of lack of information (unless the patient asks in vain for more information, or there is some danger whereby its nature or magnitude for some other reason requires to be separately taken into account by the patient in order to reach a balanced judgement) when deciding whether to submit to operation. There is no doubt that a doctor ought to draw the attention of a patient to a danger which may be special in kind or magnitude or special to the patient.

I do not subscribe to the theory that the patient is entitled to know everything, nor to the theory that doctors are entitled to decide everything. No doctor in his senses would impliedly contract at the same time to give to the patient all the information available to the doctor as a result of the doctor's training and experience and as a result of the doctor's diagnosis of the patient.

An obligation to give a patient all the information available to the doctor would often be inconsistent with the doctor's contractual obligations to have regard to the patient's best interests. Such information might confuse, other information might alarm the particular patient. Whenever the occasion arises for the doctor to tell the patient the results of the doctor's diagnosis, the possible methods of treatment and the advantages and disadvantages of the recommended treatment, the doctor must decide in the light of his training and experience and the light of his knowledge of the patient what should be said and how it should be said.

At the same time the doctor is not entitled to make the final decision with regard to treatment which may have disadvantages or dangers. Where the patient's health and future are at stake, the patient must make the final decision. The patient is free to decide whether or not to submit to the treatment recommended by the doctor and therefore the doctor impliedly contracts to provide information which is adequate to enable the patient to reach a balanced judgement, subject always to the doctor's own obligation to say nothing which the doctor is satisfied would be harmful to the patient.

If the doctor, making a balanced judgement, advises the patient to submit to the operation, the patient is entitled to reject that advice for reasons which are rational, or irrational, or for no reason. The duty of the doctor in these circumstances is to provide the patient with information which will enable the patient to make a balanced judgement if the patient chooses to make a balanced judgement. A patient may make an unbalanced judgement because he is deprived of adequate information. A patient may also make an unbalanced judgement if he is provided with too much information or is made aware of possibilities which he is not capable of assessing because of his lack of medical training, his prejudices or his personality. Thus, the provision of too much information may prejudice the attainment of the objective of restoring a patient's health.

Learning exercise   18

What does this mean for your clinical practice?

Answer to learning exercise

18   This is a seminal case in the development of informed consent. As a surgeon, you must take account of all circumstances of the case including the patient's likely reaction. Three features need to be taken into account:

1   the likelihood of a complication;
2   the severity of the effect of the complication;
3   the likely reaction of a patient who might apply undue significance to remote risks.

As a rough guide, a complication rate of less than 1% may lead to the conclusion that it is more likely to frighten the patient and put them off surgery rather than help them to make a decision. However, even this figure is not absolute and the patient who asks clearly about the risks must be given the appropriate information. The final arbiter will not be the profession but the court.

It is of interest that the question of defensive medicine is raised again and the potential effect of this problem on stifling medical progress. The same rules must apply to research and the development of new procedures. That is, the patient must be fully informed of all significant complications which may occur and are known to the practitioner. The degree of significance, as above, depends on the likelihood of the occurrence and the effect on the quality of life of the patient.

Finally, it becomes obvious that anyone obtaining informed consent must have a clear knowledge of the operative procedure to be undertaken and its likely risks and benefits. Currently it is the practice in a number of hospitals that consent is obtained by medical staff who are not the operating surgeon. This is not ideal and patients may well claim that they were not fully informed and consequently their consent was not valid. The consultant is ultimately responsible and must ensure that anyone to whom the obtaining of consent has been delegated has sufficient knowledge and understanding of the procedure to ensure the patient can form a balanced view. Complications specific to particular procedures should be specifically listed on the consent form or in the patient's notes.

Clinical case 2

You are responsible for obtaining the informed consent of Mr Adams, a patient suffering from a painful inguinal hernia. Although pleased to be undergoing surgery to relieve his condition, he is apprehensive and does not have any understanding of what a hernia is, nor of the surgery he is about to undergo.

He has previously been seen by the anaesthetist, who has passed him fit for surgery. The operation will be carried out tomorrow morning under a general anaesthetic.

You are responsible for obtaining Mr Adams' informed consent, for both the surgical procedure and the general anaesthetic.

Q1 Evaluate the link between respect for autonomy and the duty to obtain informed consent from the patient.

Q2 With examples, outline the types of information you would need to communicate to him.

Q3 How would you try to ensure that he had understood?

Clinical case 2 answers

Q1 Respect for autonomy refers to the duty to allow individuals to determine their own personal destiny, provided that they do not harm others in the process. This includes the decision to accept or reject surgical treatment on the basis of truthful information about what is being proposed, why and with what risks.

Q2 There are several essential types of information that you need to communicate:
- *The nature of his condition.* This should be described in lay terms, such as 'A hernia is the protrusion of an organ from one compartment of the body into another. An inguinal hernia is when weakness develops in certain muscles located in something called the inguinal canal, which is between the lower abdominal wall and the scrotum. When this occurs a sac of intestines pushes its way down into the scrotum.'
- *The nature of the proposed surgery.* You might say something like, 'The abdominal contents will be put back in the proper position and the defect in the abdominal wall will be repaired. When you come back from theatre you will have a dressing covering your wound which may be painful at first. Painkillers will be available should you require them. As a result of the anaesthetic, you may find you feel slightly sick and possibly you will have a headache or sore throat. This

will pass, but be sure to inform the nursing or medical staff should you begin to feel worse.'

- *Common side effects of the operation.* It is usual to mention side effects which carry a small but significant risk of occurring. In particular, the patient should be informed of the following:
    - ▼ risk of recurrence of the hernia;
    - ▼ wound neuralgia;
    - ▼ wound infection;
    - ▼ haematoma;
    - ▼ retention of urine.
- *Common side effects of the anaesthetic.* These are:
    - ▼ nausea/vomiting;
    - ▼ headache;
    - ▼ sore throat;
    - ▼ post-operative muscular aches;
    - ▼ chest infection.

Such effects will pass but the patient should be sure to inform the nursing or medical staff should they begin to feel worse. Damage to the teeth, lips, mouth and throat can also occur as a result of the insertion of a tube to help breathing while under general anaesthetic (GA). The patient will have already been seen by the anaesthetist to be passed fit for GA.

However, the surgeon obtaining consent should not assume that the patient has been informed about side effects or the importance of not eating or drinking beforehand.

As this is a healthy patient who has been seen by the anaesthetist who is happy to proceed with the operation, it is highly unlikely that any serious complications would arise. Within a healthy population undergoing a non-life-threatening elective procedure, about 1 : 100 000 patients will suffer brain damage/death as a result of the anaesthetic. The surgeon should be willing to discuss this possibility if the patient asks, trying to help the patient to put the risk into a proper perspective.

- *Consequences of no treatment.* The patient should realize that the hernia will not disappear spontaneously. Further, it may increase in size and lead to complications requiring emergency surgical procedures, for example, strangulation, which is fatal if not treated.

Q3 There are a range of possible ways to ensure that the patient understands the information provided. Always begin with the importance of maintaining empathy with the patient, trying to spot any aspects of your attempted communication that were understood with difficulty, if at all. Where there is some doubt, patients can be asked to describe in their own language their understanding of some or all of what was told to them.

The surgeon obtaining consent should always ask patients whether or not they have any questions about information which has been given, focusing specifically on areas where they have appeared not to understand. Even where patients do not admit poor understanding, if surgeons suspect it, they should go back over related details using different and simpler language themselves. Also, if written literature is available on the procedure to be undergone then it should always be offered.

Clinical case 3

Mrs Jane Henderson is a 49-year-old secondary school teacher who has had a needle biopsy of a breast lump. The histology reveals a carcinoma in her left breast. In discussing her treatment options Mrs Henderson is insistent that she will only have a lumpectomy for the removal of the tumour, stating quite clearly, 'I don't want my breast removed'. Since she is so adamant, you agree to this, against your better judgement. You obtain her written consent for this procedure but without discussing other possible treatments and risks.

One year after you perform the lumpectomy, Mrs Henderson's breast cancer returns. She sues you for battery, arguing that she did not give proper informed consent to the therapeutic lumpectomy since she had not been told about the possibility of other treatments.

Q1 Do you think that she will be successful? Why? Give examples of English case law.

Q2 Suppose she sues for negligence. Would she have any greater chance of success? Why? Give examples of English case law.

Clinical case 3 answer

Q1 No. Providing Mrs Henderson has the capacity to understand the information given to her and the information is deemed to be legally adequate, she will not be successful.

She was told of the general nature of her condition and agreed to the surgery necessary to treat it. Providing this was done, a battery will not have been committed irrespective of whether further information about alternatives and risks was communicated. Now, the most relevant case law is *Re C* (adult refusal of medical treatment, 1994).

Q2 If she could show that no further information about side effects and alternatives had been communicated then, in principle, she might win damages for negligence. However, in practice this will depend on whether or not the defendant surgeon can find expert witnesses who will testify that under the same circumstances they also would not have communicated the same information. This is because in the UK, negligence in relation to informed consent is decided by the *Bolithio* test. It does not matter whether other doctors would support the action of the defendant, but that action must be in all respects reasonable. In the majority of cases this means evidence-based, and the matter will be weighed by the court. Therefore, whether or not a defendant is guilty of negligence will depend on good practice as reflected by the majority of surgeons.

Clinical case 4

A signed consent form is not legal proof that informed consent has been given.

Q1 How does the structure and content of the form shown in Fig. 1.3.1 illustrate how this is the case?

Fig. 1.3.1

Consent form

CONSENT BY PATIENT	NOTES TO PATIENTS
Full Name:	All patients have the legal right to grant or withhold consent prior to an examination or treatment. Patients should be given sufficient information, in a way that they can understand, about the proposed treatment, risks involved and any possible alternatives.
Address:	
Postcode:	
Date of Birth:	
Please enter details or affix addressograph	Patients must also be allowed to decide whether they will agree to the treatment. They may refuse or withdraw consent at any time.
Please read this form and the notes overleaf and check that the details are correct and that you fully understand everything before signing.	
I hereby consent to undergo the operation of	Please remember:-
the nature of which has been fully explained to me. I also consent to such further or alternative operative measures as may be found necessary during the course of the operation, and to the administration of a general, local or other anaesthetic for these purposes.	The Consultant is here to help you. He/She will explain the proposed treatment/risks/alternatives to you. You may ask as many questions as you like. You can refuse treatment.
I have told the doctor about any additional procedures I would not wish to be carried out without my having the opportunity to discuss them first. These are:-	
	You may ask a relative/friend or nurse to be present.
Signed .... Patient	
Date	You have the right to seek a second opinion about your proposed treatment if you wish.
I confirm that I have explained the proposed operation, including the potential risks and any alternative options that may be considered, in terms which I believe the patient will understand.	
Signed .... Consultant	
Date	
Name of Consultant (Print)	

Clinical case 4 answer

Q1 All the form asks the surgeon obtaining consent to do, as regards providing information, is to write the name of the procedure to be undertaken. There is no space for any further details including the description of any difficulties the patient may have had in understanding the relevant information which was communicated.

Patients who sign the form might still later claim that they had not been given sufficient information to have agreed to treatment or to weigh up any associated risks. Surgeons are well advised to make a brief note of such problems as well as of the types of information which were outlined to the patient.

Clinical case 5

You are working as surgical house officer in a busy A & E department when a patient, Miss Davis, is admitted unconscious with severe injuries as the result of a road traffic accident. Soon after admission, she begins to show signs of severe internal bleeding.

Q1 Since Miss Davis is in no position to consent, are you justified in surgical intervention to try to correct her bleed? Why?

Assume that Miss Davis is conscious, says that she is a Jehovah's Witness and is carrying a Jehovah's Witness card specifically refusing a blood transfusion under any clinical circumstances.

Q2 Does she have the legal right to refuse life-saving treatment? What legal action might she successfully take out against you if you transfused her anyway? Why?

Finally, suppose instead that you were performing a dilation and curettage (D & C) under general anaesthesia and decided also to do a hysterectomy because of what you believed to be Miss Davis' malignant uterus.

Q3 Rejecting your argument that you acted in her best interest, what legal action might she successfully take against you? Why?

Clinical case 5 answers

Q1 You are justified on the grounds of 'necessity'. This is because the patient has lost her autonomy and is unable to plan her future and thus provide informed consent to surgical treatment. Morally, this is acceptable on the grounds that knowing nothing certain of the patient's own wishes you are charged with conforming to your general duty to protect life and health. It is legally acceptable for the same reason as it would be, for example, for you to intervene to save a drowning and unconscious stranger whose intent you were also unaware of.

Q2 Yes, she does have the right to refuse, provided that there is no evidence that she is being coerced by others and has not been informed of the consequences of refusal. The action would be for battery. The reason would be because you had touched her in a specific way without her permission. Indeed, she has explicitly refused such permission.

Q3 Again, the action would be for battery. Her legal (and moral) argument would be that she had only agreed to the D & C. It could not be argued that the hysterectomy was 'necessary' in the preceding sense. It was elective and could have been postponed until you awakened her from the D & C. She could then have made an informed choice.

Clinical case 6

Your patient, Mr Kelsey, is a 38-year-old diagnosed schizophrenic who is under Section 3 of the 1983 Mental Health Act. He has a form of colorectal cancer which requires immediate surgery and medical treatment.

Q1 Despite being under a section for treatment, can Mr Kelsey legally refuse consent to surgery? Why and with what moral justification?

Suppose that Mr Kelsey is severely mentally disabled and unable to consent on his own behalf.

Q2 In the UK, can his relatives consent or refuse on his behalf? Why and with what moral justification?

Q3 Who must take the decision about his treatment and with what moral and legal justification?

Clinical case 6 answers

Q1 Yes, Mr Kelsey can legally refuse provided that he is deemed competent to make an informed choice. This will depend on his ability to understand, retain, deliberate on and believe information which he is given. The moral acceptability of a sectioned patient refusing treatment under these circumstances is that the incompetence related to serious psychiatric illness entails an inability to provide informed consent for psychiatric treatment. This makes the patient vulnerable to the harm that they may cause themselves due to their illness. It does not follow from such an inability that the patient has no competence to make an informed choice about other forms of surgical treatment that may be required. Incompetence in one aspect of life should not be interpreted as incompetence in all aspects of life.

Q2 No, in the UK relatives cannot consent to or refuse treatment on behalf of others. Legally, unlike some other countries, there are no powers of guardianship here as regards consent to medical treatment. This means that one adult cannot act as a legal 'proxy' for another. Morally, the concern is that relations might not have the best interests of the patient as their primary concern. Evidence suggests that this need not be the case. On balance, since the clinician responsible for the patient's care has a professional responsibility to act for no other reason than the patient's best interests, it makes sense to give him or her the final say.

Q3 The only person who can legally provide treatment for Mr Kelsey is the clinician in charge of his care. The legal justification for this derives from the case of *F v West Berkshire Health Authority* [1989]. The moral justification rests on the argument that the clinician's duty of care entails that treatment must be provided in the best interests of the patient. No other consideration is relevant to such a decision. Therefore, because of this professional and legal responsibility, the clinician in charge is the most appropriate person to guard the patient's interests. There are examples of relatives who have acted to the contrary in clinical circumstances.

This is the voluntary permission of a patient to undergo medical treatment, and it can be withdrawn at any time. In order to give a valid consent it must be based on legally adequate information. The patient must be able to understand the nature of the proposed treatment and why it is necessary. Further they must have the capacity to make a choice based on a balance of the risks and benefits of the treatment and also have an understanding of the likely course if treatment does not take place.

The prudent patient test

The prudent patient test is used to determine what risks of medical treatment need to be discussed with the patient prior to them giving informed consent. The doctrine is based on the amount of information required by a reasonable person of sound mind and with the maturity to evaluate the options available. The material which needs to be disclosed therefore is that which, in a given set of circumstances, would be required in order to make a balanced judgement.

C ☐
S ☐
R ☐

Consent of minors

Gillick v West Norfolk and Wisbech Area Health Authority and DHSS [1986] 1 AC 112

Facts

Mrs Gillick, who at the time was the mother of four girls under the age of 16 years, wrote to her local Area Health Authority seeking assurance from them that no contraceptive advice or treatment would be given to any of her daughters while they were under 16 years of age without her knowledge or consent. The Area Health Authority refused to give such assurance and stated that, in accordance with the guidance given by the Department of Health and Social Security, the final decision on contraception pills relied upon the doctor's clinical judgement.

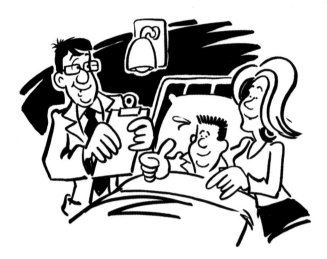

Mrs Gillick then wrote to the Health Authority stating 'I formally forbid any medical staff employed by Norfolk Area Health Authority to give any contraception, or abortion advice, or treatment whatsoever to my four daughters while they are under 16 years without my consent. Would you please acknowledge this letter and agree wholeheartedly to advise your doctors, etc. to abide by my forbidding'. There was no change in attitude of the Health Authority and therefore Mrs Gillick commenced proceedings against both the Health Authority and the Department of Health.

Learning exercise	19

What are the main issues of this case?

Answer to learning exercise

19

The issues are:

a   The rights of a parent to determine what treatment should be carried out on children who are under the age of 16 years.

b   The rights of children under the age of 16 to be treated confidentially by a medical practitioner without knowledge of their parents.

c   Whether or not a doctor who gives such advice or treatment is likely to incur criminal liability.

Excerpts from the judgement of Lord Frazer

It would appear that if the inference which Mrs Gillick's advisor seeks to draw from the provisions is justified, a minor under the age of 16 has no capacity to authorize any kind of medical advice or treatment or examination on his own body. That seems to me to be so surprising that I cannot accept it in the absence of clear provision to that effect. It seems to be verging on the absurd to suggest that a girl or boy aged 15 could not effectively consent, for example, to have a medical examination of some trivial injury to his body or even to have a broken arm set.

Of course the consent of the parents should normally be asked, but they may not be immediately available. Provided the patient, whether a boy or a girl, is capable of understanding what is proposed, and expressing his or her own wishes, I see no good reason for holding that he or she lacks the capacity to express vividly and effectively and to authorize the medical man to make the examination or give treatment which he advises. After all, a minor under the age of 16 can, within certain limits, enter into a contract, he or she can also sue and be sued and can give evidence on oath. Moreover, a girl under 16 can give sufficient effective consent to sexual intercourse to lead to the legal result that the man involved does not commit the crime of rape.

Accordingly, I am not disposed to hold now, for the first time, that a girl aged less than 16 lacks the power to give valid consent to contraceptive advice or treatment, merely on account of her age.

It was, I think, accepted by both Mrs Gillick and the Department of Health and Social Services and in any event I hold, that parental rights to control a child do not exist for the benefit of the parent. They exist for the benefit of the child and they are justified only insofar as they enable the parent to perform his duties towards the child, and towards other children and family.

The solution depends on a judgement on what is best for the welfare of the child. Nobody doubts that in the overwhelming majority of cases, the best judge of a child's welfare is his or her parents; that is why it would and should be most unusual for a doctor to advise a child without the knowledge or consent of the parents on contraceptive matters. But, as I have already pointed out, Mrs Gillick has to go further if she was to obtain the first declaration that she seeks. She has to justify the absolute right of a parent. But there may be circumstances in which the doctor is a better judge of the medical advice and treatment which will conduce to a girl's welfare than her parents. It is notorious that children of both sexes are often reluctant to confide in their parents about sexual matters.

The doctor will, in my opinion, be justified in proceeding without a parent's consent or even their knowledge providing he is satisfied on the following matters:

1 That a girl (although under 16 years of age) will understand his advice.
2 That he cannot persuade her to inform her parents or allow him to inform the parents that she is seeking contraceptive advice.
3 That she is very likely to be or continue having sexual intercourse with or without contraceptive treatment.
4 That unless she receives contraceptive advice or treatment her physical and mental health or both are likely to suffer.
5 That her best interests require him to give her contraceptive advice and treatment or both without parental consent.

That result ought not to be regarded as a licence for doctors to disregard the wishes of parents on this matter whenever they find it convenient to do so. Any doctor who behaves in such a way would be failing to discharge his professional responsibilities, and I would expect him to be disciplined by his own professional body accordingly.

This appeal is concerned with doctors who honestly intend to act with the best interests of the girl, and I think it unlikely that a doctor who gives contraceptive advice or treatment with that intention would commit an offence.

Per *Lord Scarman*

Blackstone accepts that by statute and by case law the varying ages of discretion have been fixed for various purposes. But it is clear that this was done to achieve certainty where it was considered necessary and in no way limits the principle that parental right endures only so long as is needed for the protection of the child.

The House must, in my view, be understood as having accepted that, save where statute otherwise provides, a minor's capacity to make his or her own decision depends on the minor having sufficient understanding and intelligence to make the decision and is not to be determined by reference to any judicially fixed age limit.

[In the case of contraception] it is not enough that she should understand the nature of the advice being given but she must also have sufficient maturity to understand what is involved. There are moral and family questions, especially her relationship with her parents; long-term problems associated with the emotional impact of pregnancy and termination; and the risks to health of having sexual intercourse at her age, risks which contraception may diminish but cannot eliminate. It is possible that a doctor may satisfy himself that she is able to appraise these factors before he can safely proceed on the basis that she has in law the capacity to consent to contraceptive treatment.

Learning exercise	20
What does this mean for your clinical practice?	

Answer to learning exercise

20　Notwithstanding that this case involves discussion of contraceptive facilities, those under the age of 16 have the legal capacity to consent to medical examination and treatment if they have sufficient maturity and intelligence to understand the nature and implications of proposed treatment. It was specifically mentioned by Lord Templeman that this included that a doctor may remove tonsils or a troublesome appendix with the consent of an intelligent boy or girl under 15 and the doctor would be well advised to discuss the matter with the child as well as the parents, who do not have overriding control. This may also apply to other procedures such as plastic surgery, for example operations on bat ears or to alter the shape of the nose.

A parent's right to control a minor child is a dwindling right and exists only insofar as is required for the child's benefit and protection. This is not by reference to a fixed age but depends on the degree of intelligence and understanding of a particular child. The bona fide exercise of a doctor's own clinical judgement as to what they honestly believe to be necessary for the physical, mental and emotional health of the child will not lead to commission of a criminal offence.

Therefore, a minor has a right to consent to treatment if they are 'Gillick mature' and this cannot be overridden with parental responsibility. However, the court retains the power to override such consent if it comes to the conclusion that this would be in the best interests of the child.

Note that the same is not true for refusal of treatment. A minor has no such absolute right. Parents, or those with parental responsibility, may override the minor's refusal and a doctor is therefore authorized to proceed according to his or her clinical judgement. If both the minor and those with parental responsibility refuse consent, then the court may still take the final decision in the interests of the child.

Clinical case 7

You are a paediatric surgeon asked to place a Hickman line in an 11-year-old cancer patient undergoing bone marrow transplantation. The child, Lucy Lawrence, has already had two courses of chemotherapy and experienced uncommonly distressing side effects from the last. The chances of the transplantation succeeding are not great.

Q1 How and from whom would you obtain informed consent to insert the Hickman line? With what moral and legal justification?

Q2 Outline Lucy's moral and legal rights, if any, in this situation. Suppose that Lucy refused to give you permission to insert the line. What course of action would you advise and how would you morally and legally defend it?

Clinical case 7 answers

Q1 You should obtain informed consent from Lucy's parents. The legal justification is that according to the 1969 Family Law Reform Act, 16 is the age of consent for surgical treatment. Under that age, it should ordinarily be provided by parents or by those with parental responsibility. The moral justification is that young people may not have the competence to act in their own best interests as regards surgical treatment. If they make choices based more on immediate preference than on serious deliberation, they may foreclose later opportunities to exercise a more competent choice. In the case of Lucy, the choice to refuse treatment (if, for her, it is wrong) would presumably lead to her death.

Q2 Notwithstanding the above, Lucy does have rights pertaining to informed consent. According to the 1989 Children Act, she has the right to be consulted and to have her views about future treatment taken into account. This is not something that is discretionary. It has to be done to the degree that her competence will permit it and these views noted (*Gillick* maturity).

Morally, this is justified by the fact that although age may have limited her autonomy, Lucy is still the person who will have to bear the consequences of a distressing treatment. To inflict it on her without as much consultation as is practicably possible would be just as immoral as doing so on adults without obtaining their informed consent. It is, after all, Lucy's body and not her parents'.

The response to Lucy's refusal should be dictated by the content of her wishes, along with her competence and understanding of her situation. Assuming that, as is often the case, her understanding is good, the appropriate course of action is not immediately to treat. Rather, attempts should be made for the parents and health-care team themselves fully to understand why Lucy is refusing. Parents should be

C ☐
S ☐
R ☐

strongly encouraged to comply with her wishes, especially if her prognosis is poor. Yet with recent case law in mind, it should be remembered that Lucy does not have the strict right to refuse treatment deemed to be life-saving until she is 18.

Persistent vegetative state

Airedale NHS Trust v Bland [1993] 1 FLR 1026

Facts

At the age of 17 and a half, Anthony Bland was injured in the Hillsborough Football Ground disaster as a result of which he sustained catastrophic and irreversible brain damage which left him in a persistent vegetative state (PVS). His brainstem remained alive so he could breathe unaided, his digestion continued, but he had no cognitive function at all. In the eyes of the medical world and of the law a person is not clinically dead as long as the brainstem retains its function, which it was doing.

In order to maintain him, feeding and hydration were achieved artificially by means of a nasogastric tube and excretory functions regulated by a catheter and by enemas. From time to time he would have chest and urinary tract infections which were treated by antibiotics. The undisputed consensus of medical opinion was that there was no prospect whatsoever that he would make a recovery but there was every likelihood he would maintain his present status of existence for many years providing the medical care which he was receiving was continued. At no time before the disaster had he given any indication of his wishes if such a situation should arise, but his father said in evidence that his son 'would not want to live like that'. The Trust, the parents and the consultant in charge applied to the court for direction.

Learning exercise	21

What are the main issues of this case?

Answer to learning exercise

21 The main issues are:

 a In what circumstances, if any, can those having a duty to feed an invalid lawfully stop doing so?

 b Under the law as it now stands, would those withdrawing the treatment be committing a criminal offence and particularly the offence of murder?

Excerpts from the judgement of Lord Keith

The first point being that it is unlawful, so as to constitute both a tort and the crime of battery, to administer treatment to an adult who is conscious and of sound mind without his consent. Such a person is completely at liberty to decline to undergo treatment, even if the result of his doing so will be that he will die. This extends to the situation where the person, in the anticipation of this, through one cause or another entering into a condition such as PVS, gives clear instructions that in such an event he is not to be given medical care, including artificial feeding, designed to keep him alive.

The second point is that it very commonly occurs that a person due to an accident or some other cause becomes unconscious and thus not able to give or withhold consent to medical treatment. In that situation it is lawful, under the principle of necessity, for medical men to apply such treatment as in their informed opinion is in the best interests of the unconscious patient. That is what happened in the case of Anthony Bland when he was first dealt with by the emergency services and later taken to hospital.

The object of medical treatment and care is to benefit the patient. It may do so by taking steps to prevent the occurrence of illness, or, if any illness does occur, by taking steps towards curing it. Where an illness or the effects of an injury cannot be cured, then efforts are directed towards preventing deterioration or relieving pain and suffering. Sound medical opinion takes the view that if a PVS patient shows no sign of recovery after 6 months, or at most a year, then there is no prospect whatever of any recovery. There are techniques available to make it possible to ascertain the state of the cerebral cortex, and in Anthony Bland's case, these indicate that, as mentioned above, it degenerated into a mass of watery fluid. The fundamental question then comes to be whether continuance of the present regime of treatment and care, more than 3 years after the injuries that resulted in PVS, would confirm any benefit.

In *Re F* (mental patient; sterilization) this House held that it would be lawful to sterilize a female mental patient who was incapable of giving consent for this procedure. The ground of the decision was that sterilization would be in the patient's best interest because her life would be fuller and more agreeable if she was sterilized than if she were not. In *Re J* (a minor) the Court of Appeal held it to be lawful to withhold life-saving treatment from a very young child in circumstances where the child's life, if saved, would be one irredeemably racked by pain and agony.

In both cases it was possible to make a value judgement as to the consequences to a sensate being, in one case, withholding and the other case, administering the treatment in question. In the case of a permanently insensate being, who if continuing to live would never experience the slightest actual discomfort, it is difficult, if not impossible, to make any relevant comparison between continued existence and the absence of it. It is, however, perhaps permissible to say that to an individual with no cognitive capacity whatsoever, and no prospect of ever recovering any such capacity in this world, it must be a matter of complete indifference whether he lives or dies. For once an individual has assumed responsibility for the care of another who cannot look after himself or herself, whether as a medical practitioner or otherwise, that responsibility cannot lawfully be shed unless arrangements are being made for the responsibility to be taken over by someone else.

It is, of course, true that in general it would not be lawful for a medical practitioner who assumed responsibility for the care of an unconscious patient simply to give up treatment in circumstances where continuance of it would confer some benefit on the patient. On the other hand, a medical practitioner is under no duty to continue to treat such a patient where a large volume of informed and responsible medical opinion is to the effect that no benefit at all would be confirmed by continuance.

[Therefore] the principle is not an absolute one. It does not compel a medical practitioner on pain of criminal sanction to treat a patient who will die if he does not, contrary to the express wishes of the patient. It does not authorize forcible feeding of prisoners on hunger strike. It does not compel the temporary keeping alive of patients who are terminally ill where to do so would merely prolong their suffering. On the other hand, it forbids the taking of active measures to cut short the life of a terminally ill patient. In my judgement it does no violence to the principle to hold that it is lawful to cease to give medical treatment and care to a PVS patient who has been in that state for over 3 years, considering that to do so involves invasive manipulation of the patient's body to which he has not consented and which confers no benefit upon him.

Per *Lord Goff*

I must, however, stress, at this point, that the law draws a crucial distinction between cases in which a doctor decides not to provide, or to continue to provide, for his patient treatment or care which could or might prolong his life and those in which he decides, for example by administering a lethal drug, actively to bring his patient's life to an end. As I have already indicated, the former may be lawful, either because the doctor is giving effect to the patient's wishes by withholding the treatment or care or even in certain circumstances in which a patient is incapacitated from stating whether or not he gives his consent. But it is not lawful for a doctor to administer a drug to his patient to bring about his death even though that course is prompted by a humanitarian desire to end his suffering, however great that suffering may be. So to act is to cross the Rubicon which runs between on the one hand the care of the living patient and on the other hand euthanasia—actively causing his death to avoid or end his suffering. Euthanasia is not lawful at common law. The law does not feel able to authorize euthanasia, even in circumstances such as these; for once euthanasia is recognized as lawful in these circumstances, it is difficult to see any logical basis for excluding it in others.

I return to the patient who, because of unsound mind or having been rendered unconscious by accident or illness, is incapable of stating whether or not he consents to treatment or care. In such circumstances, it is now established that a doctor may lawfully treat such a patient if he acts in his best interests, and indeed that, if the patient is already in his care, he is under a duty to treat him. For my part I can see no reason why, as a matter of principle, a decision by a doctor whether or not to initiate or continue to provide, treatment or care which could or might have the effect to prolong such a patient's life should not be governed by the same fundamental principle. Of course, in the great majority of cases, the best interests of the patients are likely to require that treatment of this kind, if available, should be given to the patient. But this may not always be so. To take a simple example it cannot be right that a doctor, who has under his care a patient who is suffering painfully from terminal cancer, should be under an absolute obligation to perform upon him major surgery to abate another condition which, if unabated, would or might shorten his life still further. The doctor who is caring for such a patient cannot, in my opinion, be under an absolute obligation to prolong his life by any means available to him, regardless of the quality of the patient's life. Common humanity requires otherwise, as do medical ethics and good medical practice accepted in this country and overseas.

Guidance for a case such as the present is to be found in a discussion paper on treatment of patients in PVS, issued in September 1992 by the Medical Ethics Committee of the British Medical Association. There are four safeguards:

1 Every effort should be made at rehabilitation for at least 6 months after the injury.

2 The diagnosis of irreversible PVS should not be confirmed until at least 12 months

after the injury, with the effect that any decision to withhold life-prolonging treatment will be delayed for that period.

3 The diagnosis should be agreed by two other independent doctors.

4 Generally, the wishes of the patient's immediate family should be given great weight.

The committee is firmly of the opinion that the relatives cannot be determinative of the treatment. Indeed, if that were not so, the relatives would be able to dictate to the doctor what is in the best interests of the patient, which cannot be right. Even so, a decision to withhold life-prolonging treatment, such as artificial feeding, must require close co-operation with those close to the patient. It is recognized, that in practice, their views and the opinions of doctors will coincide in many cases.

I find to the extent to which doctors should, as a matter of practice, seek the guidance of the court, by way of an application for declaratory relief before withholding life-prolonging treatment from a PVS patient.

For the respondents, Mr Francis suggested that an adequate safeguard would be provided if reference to the court required certain specific circumstances, i.e. where there was known to be a medical disagreement as to the diagnosis and prognosis, and problems had arisen with the patient's relatives—disagreement by the next of kin with the medical recommendations; actual or apparent conflict of interest between the next of kin and the patient; dispute between members of the patient's family; or absence of any next of kin to give their consent.

There is, I consider, much to be said for the view that an application to the court will not be needed in every case, but only in particular circumstances such as those suggested by Mr Francis.

It is not to be forgotten, moreover, that doctors who for conscious reasons would feel unable to discontinue life support in such circumstances can presumably, like those who have a conscientious objection to abortion, abstain from involvement in such work.

Per *Lord Browne-Wilkinson*

The crux is the extent of the duty owed by a hospital and a doctor to Anthony Bland. In order to analyse the nature of that duty, it is necessary first to consider the relationship between a doctor and a patient who, through mental disability, is unable to consent to treatment. Any treatment given by a doctor to a patient which is invasive (i.e. involves any interference with the physical integrity of the patient) is unlawful unless done with the consent of the patient—it constitutes the crime of battery and the tort of trespass to the person. Thus, in the case of an adult who is mentally competent, the artificial feeding regime, and the attendant steps to evacuate the contents of the bladder, would be unlawful unless the patient consented to it. A mentally competent patient can at any time put an end to life-support systems by refusing his consent for their continuation. In the ordinary case of murder by a positive act of commission, the consent of the victim is no defence. But where the charge is one of murder by omission to do an act and the act omitted could only be done with the consent of the patient, refusal by the patient of consent to the doing of such acts, does, indirectly, provide a defence to the charge of murder. The doctor cannot owe to the patient any duty to maintain his life where that life can only be sustained by intrusive medical care to which the patient cannot consent.

▼

How then does the matter stand in the case of a patient who, by reason of his being under age, or like Anthony Bland, of full age but mentally disabled, is unable to give consent to treatment? So far as minors are concerned, the guardian of the child can consent, failing which the court exercising the Crown's rights under wardship jurisdiction can consent on the child's behalf. Until 1960, the court had the same jurisdiction over adults who were mentally incompetent. But, by the joint effect of the Mental Health Act 1959 and the revocation of the Warrant under the *Sign Manual* under which the jurisdiction of the Crown over those of unsound mind was conferred on the courts, the courts ceased to have jurisdiction over the person of a mentally incompetent adult. As a result, the court even if it thought fit, has no power on Anthony Bland's behalf either to consent or refuse consent to the continuation of invasive procedures involved in artificial feeding.

Faced with this lacuna in the law, the House in *Re F* developed and laid down a principle, based on the concept of necessity, by which a doctor can lawfully treat a patient who cannot consent to such treatment if it is in the best interests of the patient to receive such treatment. In my view, the correct answer in the present case depends on the extent of the right to continue lawfully to invade the bodily integrity of Anthony Bland without his consent. If in the circumstances they [the doctors] have no right to continue artificial feeding, they cannot be in breach of any duty by ceasing to provide such feeding.

Finally, the conclusion I have reached would appear to some to be almost irrational. How can it be lawful to allow a patient to die slowly, though painlessly, over a period of weeks from lack of food but unlawful to produce his immediate death by lethal injection, thereby saving his family from yet another ordeal to add to the tragedy that has already struck them? I find it difficult to find a moral answer to that question. But it is undoubtedly the law and nothing I have said casts doubt on the proposition that the doing of a positive act with the intention of ending life is and remains a murder.

Learning exercise   22

What does this mean for your clinical practice?

Answer to learning exercise

22   A patient who is of sound mind has an absolute right to decide whether he will or will not accept treatment, and a doctor would be committing an assault if in any way they invaded the patient, for example by taking blood or inserting a drip, without specific consent. In the case of children, consent may be given or withheld by the parents subject to the previous case of *Gillick* with the final arbiter being the Court.

However the Court has no such jurisdiction over the body of a mentally disabled adult. In this case a doctor can lawfully treat a patient who cannot consent to treatment if it is in the best interests of the patient to receive such treatment. The doctor's decision is assessed by reference to a decision in accordance with a practice accepted at the time by a responsible body of medical opinion (*Bolam* and *Bolithio*, see above). There is no requirement for a doctor to continue life support for a patient in a PVS, as set out in four safeguards laid down by the Medical Ethics Committee of the British Medical Association which are:

- Every effort should be made for 6 months after the injury.
- The diagnosis of irreversible PVS should not be considered confirmed until at least 12 months after the injury with the effect that any decision to withhold life or prolong treatment will be delayed for that period.
- The diagnosis should be agreed by two other independent doctors.
- Generally the wishes of the patient's immediate family would be given great weight.

   If there is a known medical disagreement as to the diagnosis and prognosis, or if there are problems with the relatives as stated above, then doctors would be well advised in each case to apply to the court for a declaration as to the legality of any proposed discontinuance of life support.

Euthanasia

R v Adams [1957] Crim LR 365

Facts

Mrs Morrell, an elderly woman aged 81 years, died in 1950. She had been a patient of Dr Adams for 2 years. He prescribed increasing quantities of drugs, particularly heroin and morphia, and eventually paraldehyde. Mrs Morrell died having apparently been in a coma for the last days of her life. By Mrs Morrell's last will, made approximately 3 months before she died, Dr Adams knew he was to receive an old chest containing silver and also, if her son predeceased her, a Rolls-Royce car. The following month Mrs Morrell made a codicil to her will, excluding Dr Adams from it completely. Following her death, Dr Adams did, in fact, receive the chest and the Rolls-Royce car, not because he was a beneficiary under the last will but as an act of favour by Mr Morrell, the lady's son.

During the trial, one of the nurses involved stated that, relying on her memory of what happened 6 or 7 years ago, by the time Dr Adams gave his injections the patient was very dopey and half asleep. She was weaker in every way, and when she last saw her, 11 days before death, Mrs Morrell was 'almost semiconscious and rambling'. She added she saw no real signs of pain.

Learning exercise	23

What are the main issues of this case?

C ☐
S ☐
R ☐

Answer to learning exercise

23 The main issues are:

   a Did the injections of morphine and heroin, combined with the paraldehyde at the end, hasten death?

   b Was Dr Adams justified in prescribing such doses?

   c Was it wise for him to accept gifts from his patient since he knew about the will before her death?

Comments

This case did not come to appeal but was halted after 17 days with John Bodkin Adams acquitted of the murder of Mrs Morrell.

A number of issues are raised pertaining to good medical practice. The first is the principle of dual action. Any drug has more than one effect. As stated in the case of Anthony Bland (see above), giving an injection with a specific intention of ending life, i.e. euthanasia, is illegal and would lead to a charge of murder. However, if the first purpose of medicine, the restoration of health, could no longer be achieved, there is still much for a doctor to do in a terminal case. He is entitled to do all that is proper and necessary to relieve pain and suffering even if the measures taken might incidentally shorten life by hours or perhaps even longer.

In summing up, Judge Devlin stated that a doctor who decided whether or not to administer the drug could not do his job if he was thinking in terms of hours or months of life. He pointed out the defence in the present case was that the treatment given by Dr Adams was designed to promote comfort, and if it was right and proper treatment, the fact that it shortened life did not convict him of murder.

Second, the barrister for the defence produced a number of exercise books which contained the actual nursing records. The nurse stated that as far as her memory served her, Mrs Morrell was dopey and half asleep, almost semiconscious and rambling. The entry for that day showed that Mrs Morrell's lunch consisted of 'partridge, celery, pudding and brandy and soda'. The entry by a second nurse on 12 November, the day before Mrs Morrell died, stated that the patient was 'awake' but quiet. This obviously casts doubt on the contention that Dr Adams was giving drugs to end life and had put her into a coma for many days. The important feature here was the presence of contemporaneous records so that the witness did not have to rely on memory after a number of years.

Third, one of the actions which led to the establishment of a motive for murder was his acceptance of gifts from his patient, including the chest of silverware and a Roll-Royce car. In the event, that part of the will had been withdrawn 2 months before she died, but it nevertheless opened the doctor to accusations that he had ulterior motives.

Learning exercise	24

What does this mean for your clinical practice?

Answer to learning exercise

24 Clearly a medical practitioner has to be very careful and be clear in his mind as to the reason why a particular course of action, including drug therapy, is contemplated. This must be to the benefit of the patient. From the *Bland* case, we know that it is acceptable under the circumstances as laid down to withdraw medical treatment, but the giving of drugs is a positive act as opposed to an act of omission. If the intention is euthanasia, i.e. to cause the early death of a patient, rather than render him or her more comfortable, then a doctor would be open to the charge of murder.

Contemporary records proved to be of vital importance in Dr Adams' defence. Relying on memory of events that happened 6 years ago can lead to a lot of dispute. Therefore, you should make sure your notes are detailed, accurate and written at the time.

Finally, a relationship of trust is assumed between a doctor and his patient. This is not just personal but it is best to avoid situations, such as receiving gifts, which may give the impression to others of an ulterior motive. In general terms, it would be wise to make sure that any gift, whether it be from a patient or from a drug company (for example, hospitality), is not of high value in financial terms.

Whistle-blowing

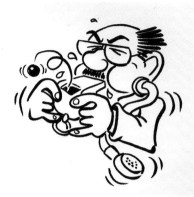

There have been several high-profile cases where it has been suggested that standards of care fell below an acceptable level and that other practitioners knew it was happening but did nothing to stop it. Indeed, in one recent instance, when a junior member of staff attempted to bring his concerns to senior staff it would appear that not only was he not listened to but he also found difficulty in finding further employment.

To date, these cases have basically raised ethical issues and have not been tested in court. Nevertheless there are some legal precedents, which suggest that under such circumstances a claim against Trust and medical staff for negligence may be substantiated.

Donoghue v Stevenson [1932] AC 562

Facts

Mrs Donoghue was taken to a cafe and a friend bought her a ginger beer. The bottle was opaque. Mrs Donoghue drank some of the ginger beer but when she poured out the rest a decomposing snail fell out of the bottle. She became ill and sued the manufacturer for negligence.

Learning exercise	25
What is the classic triad for legal negligence?	

Answer to learning exercise

25   The classic triad is duty, breach and damage. In this case, the difficulty as the law stood in 1932 was establishing that the manufacturer had a duty of care towards Mrs Donoghue.

Learning exercise   26

In medical cases, what name is given to the special relationship between a doctor and patient?

Answer to learning exercise

26   The special relationship between a patient and doctor is termed a fiduciary relationship.

Excerpt from the judgement of Lord Atkin

The rule that you are to love your neighbour becomes in law, 'you must not injure your neighbour' and the lawyers' question, 'who is my neighbour?' receives a restricted reply. You must take reasonable care to avoid acts or omissions that you can reasonably foresee would be likely to injure your neighbour. Who then, in law, is my neighbour? The answer seems to be persons who are so closely and directly affected by my act that they ought reasonably to have them in contemplation as being so affected when I am directing my mind to the acts or omissions which are called into question.

Learning exercise   27

What does this mean for your clinical practice?

Answer to learning exercise

27   You have the privilege of being a medical practitioner. There is therefore a very special relationship between you and any patient with whom you come in contact. Note that this does not simply include patients directly under your care.

Under normal circumstances the law draws a distinction between the infliction of harm through a positive action and merely allowing harm to occur by failing to prevent it. Pure omissions do not normally give rise to a liability in negligence because no duty of care arises. However, there are two main exceptions that affect you directly:

- Where you undertake to perform a task, then you have assumed a duty to carry out that task carefully (see *Barnett v The Chelsea and Kensington Hospital*, p. 119).
- Where there is a fiduciary relationship. This comes from the case of *Stansbie v Troman* [1948] 2 KB 48, where the defendant, who was a decorator, left the plaintiff's house without locking up and the house was burgled. In other words there was a duty of care, it was breached and as a result damage occurred.

You have a duty to make sure that as far as possible patients are treated properly and do not come to any harm. Although it has not as yet been tested in court, the likelihood is that cases such as those cited above would be used as a basis of a claim in negligence against a doctor who did not report concerns to the appropriate authority. You should therefore discuss your concerns with senior medical staff. It would of course depend on the situation but these people may be your educational supervisor, another consultant usually in the same speciality, the lead clinician or the medical director.

Do not be afraid to ask questions about the management of any case with which you are involved. You are a trainee and no consultant with whom you are working should object to such a discussion, and indeed this should be positively encouraged. If you find that there is a problem discussing cases then you should not hesitate to discuss the matter with your educational supervisor or the department of your postgraduate dean who is responsible for the training posts.

Refer back to Clinical case 1, which deals with confidentiality.

Comment

Every individual owes what is termed a duty of care towards their neighbour. Your neighbour is someone who is 'so closely and directly affected by my act that I ought reasonably to have them in contemplation as being so affected when I am directing my mind to the acts or omissions which are called in question'. (*Donoghue v Stevenson [1932]*; see p. 143). Pure omissions do not normally give rise to liability except where a person undertakes to perform a task, when that person assumes a duty to act carefully in carrying it out, or where there is a special relationship in existence, such as between a doctor and patient. Any doctor at any level of seniority is therefore obliged to take action when he feels that an action or omission by another (be it a doctor or trust management) is liable to harm a patient.

C ☐
S ☐
R ☐

Authorship of scientific papers

It is an ethical obligation on any person whose name appears as an author to a scientific paper to ensure that they have participated fully in the study. This includes participation in the design of the study, collection and assessment of data, and participation in the manuscript preparation. Each author has to assume full responsibility for the content of the paper. Individuals whose contributions fall short of these exacting criteria should be credited in the acknowledgements at the end of the paper. Other individuals whose contributions were confined to contributions that were part of their normal remunerated position, such as secretarial or technical assistance, do not normally require formal acknowledgement.

Clinical case 8

You have started a research position in the academic department of surgery. You have been asked to review several patients to complete a prospective study on the outcome of a new surgical technique. Your results from this subset are not as promising as those from the earlier patients reviewed by your senior colleague, who had undertaken the procedures himself.

Later when the manuscript has been prepared for submission, you note that your results have been altered to a more favourable outcome. When you tackle the surgeon about the data change, he claims that your inexperience had led you to misinterpret the outcomes. He presses you to sign the 'letter of transmittal' to the journal and enquires about your search for a specialist registrar position and asks who is providing references for you.

Q1 What is the appropriate action for you to take?

Clinical case 8 answer

Q1 Duty of care has been discussed in the clinical context. Here, it is extended to the field of research.

Personal integrity, once lost, can never be fully recovered. Unfortunately there have been a few recent cases where a scientist's personal ambition has been such that they were prepared to compromise their integrity to achieve their aims. You must never contemplate such a course of action and must not allow yourself to be associated with others who do.

In this case, there would appear to be a loosely veiled threat to career progress. You must resist the threat and immediately discuss all the issues with your head of department, bringing any evidence you have, such as your original results and those which appear to be altered. If the head of department is himself compromised, you should discuss the matter with the head of another academic department or the head of the ethics committee.

Be assured that very few members of academic departments would involve themselves in any way with such practice and will guide and assist you in bringing such practices to light. Remember, those who have been guilty of such behaviour have been publicly exposed and in serious cases have been forced to resign from very senior positions. Maintain your integrity at all costs throughout your career and do not compromise your position in the slightest, even if it would appear initially to give some short-term advantage to your career.

Risk management

All medical interventions carry an element of risk, by which is meant an outcome below that which was intended. It may actually place a patient in a worse position than they were before treatment commenced. Risk management requires that the chances of such an occurrence are minimized, and when they do happen actions are taken to review what happened, to learn any lessons, and where necessary to change practice to minimize the likelihood of any recurrence. This requires self-reflection, honesty and a robust system of audit of professional practice on an ongoing basis.

The concept of clinical freedom

You have now covered the basics of law and ethics as applied to clinical practice. So where does this leave doctors and their freedom to exercise clinical judgement? Our society grants rights to individuals, not least of which is the right to decide whether or not a particular course of action is in their best interests, and to accept or reject those which in their opinion, however flawed, may harm them either physically or psychologically.

Clinical freedom is, in fact, freedom at an intellectual level. Medicine moves forwards at an ever-increasing rate and no practitioner can afford to stand still in terms of knowledge or competence. You must continually strive to keep up to date, and any changes in practice should be supported by a logical analysis of the literature, in other words evidence-based medicine.

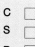

C ☐
S ☐
R ☐

Further, as medicine advances, knowledge and technology are becoming very complex and sophisticated. This requires teamwork, both between clinicians and between clinicians and management, who have a duty to provide the appropriate conditions and financial resources in order to deliver a quality service for patients. All teams need some form of control and leadership, and hence the necessity for clinical governance, which may be defined as corporate responsibility for clinical practice.

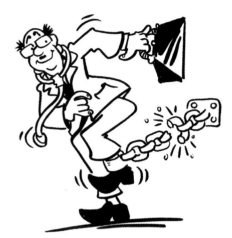

Clinical freedom is therefore freedom within bounds. Rather like most sports, there are rules and regulations laid down by a governing body, which may consist of players, spectators and, indeed, society at large, especially if there is any question of physical harm. If a player wishes to participate in a particular game such as football, then he must agree to abide by the rules, which are policed by the match officials. Within the game, players may assume many different positions, from attacker to defender, from centre forward to goal keeper, and may with advantage be as innovative as possible.

Therefore, players enjoy a great freedom on the field of play as long as they stay within the rules. If they do not, there will be sanctions, and, in extreme cases, expulsion from the sport.

This analogy obviously carries over into the field of medicine. The boundaries are set by the law, the profession and society. Within the boundaries, however, doctors are asked to display their talents to the full, both as individuals and in teams, with the ultimate goal of providing a quality service.

Staying within bounds is not difficult. Simply treat others with the respect and professionalism which you would expect to be shown towards yourself or your family and you will not go far wrong.

Clinical governance

This judgement is at the heart of the issues of clinical governance, which has been defined as corporate responsibility for clinical practice. This is basically a quality issue and it is a means whereby trust management can ensure that staff are adequately trained and are continually updated. It recognizes that the delivery of medical care requires a team approach. The outcomes are determined not only by those individuals directly caring for the patient, but also by others in a service capacity as well as the level of

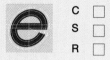

C ☐
S ☐
R ☐

resources made available. It therefore forms a link between the management of the Health Service and the hands-on practitioners, and makes the chief executive of a trust directly responsible for the quality of the clinical care. There is a need for a system whereby good practice and evidence-based innovations can be systemically disseminated and implemented.

Summary

In this Unit you have read about the need for society to have legal rules to govern behaviour, the basis for those rules, and the need for rules to govern medical practice. Topics explored included duty of care, standards of care, level of knowledge and competence, and issues surrounding confidentiality. You then covered negligence and how it is defined, consent, informed consent, dealing with minors, persistent vegetative state, end of life issues and whistle-blowing.

Planned care: patient preparation

Authors

N. Appleyard

D. Bryden

N. Edwards

S. Fletcher

G. W. G. French

J. B. Groves

G. Howell

D. Howlett

M. Larvin

J. Macfie

Introduction

Foundation Year 1 focuses on routine patient care. This does not mean that you will not be looking after emergency admissions, nor that you will not be faced with acute problems in electively admitted patients! You will find that the principles of planned care as covered in STEP™ Foundation Modules 1 and 2 are also useful in your later learning in the second Foundation year, when you will gain confidence with acute care.

This is a Unit that you should work through in full, and will cover the management of patients up to the point of their planned procedure. Module 2: Next STEP™ will cover the management of everything following a patient's planned procedure

This Unit looks at the general principles of preparing patients for planned admission. It will cover risk assessment, investigations and prophylaxis against common post-procedural complications. Although the emphasis is on planned surgery, exactly the same principles apply to other less invasive procedures such as endoscopy, radiological interventions and certain pathology testing such as endocrine assessments.

STEP™ Foundation user guide

Work steadily and identify topics that require more work—use a highlighter if you wish, and scribble notes and comments in the wide margins provided. Add links to other useful resources you discover. This will all help you to revise later.

For efficient study, use the tick boxes at the end of each section, writing a date alongside. This will remind you when you have:

- **C** Completed your reading
- **S** Self-assessed using *e*STEP™ Foundation website
- **R** Revised

Do remember to log in to *e*STEP™ Foundation regularly. *e*STEP™ Foundation contains a rich variety of supporting material to make your study more efficient. *e*STEP™ Foundation is updated frequently and will contain late-breaking amendments, unit by unit, as well as valuable additional resources.

 Surgery journal

 eSTEP™ resource

 Textbook

 Weblink

We hope you enjoy working through this Unit. Please use *e*STEP™ Foundation website to provide us with feedback and any comments or suggestions.

Expected learning outcomes

When you have completed this Unit, you will be able to:

- carry out your role effectively in the preparation of patients for planned procedures
- identify the potential problems which may occur preoperatively in patients with intercurrent disease
- organize investigations for your patients, taking into consideration the procedure planned and the health of the individual patient
- exchange useful information with the anaesthetist before the day of the procedure based on your understanding of basic principles of sedation and anaesthesia
- refer patients appropriately for specialist advice (including to the anaesthetist) for optimization of their intercurrent conditions
- apply the currently available scoring systems to help you weigh up the risks for these individuals
- contribute significantly to the reduction of clinical risk, improved patient experience and also to the efficient functioning of your hospital.

Clinical topics

Clinical topics

Principles of planned care

Pre-admission preparation

Financial constraints in the UK National Health Service and health-care systems around the world have made it essential that all hospitals use their limited budgets in the most efficient and cost-effective way possible. It has been estimated that about half the adult patients scheduled for a planned procedure have some sort of coexisting disease, unrelated to the presenting condition. This problem is increased in the elderly. Nevertheless, it used to be common practice for patients undergoing routine elective surgery to be admitted to the ward barely a few hours before the operating list is scheduled to start.

It is a major problem when a patient, who is admitted at such short notice, is found to be insufficiently worked up or deemed to be unfit for surgery. There is not usually enough time to improve that patient's condition sufficiently to make it safe to operate on the same day. It is then too short a notice to arrange another suitably starved and prepared patient to be admitted from the waiting list. Precious bed space is used up and valuable operating time is lost. This lost time can never be made up! The same constraints apply to patients scheduled for endoscopic, radiological or other non-surgical procedures.

To avoid this scenario and to ensure that the sequence of admission, procedure, recovery and discharge runs smoothly, most departments run a pre-admission assessment clinic where patients are seen about 3 weeks ahead of their planned admission. Unfortunately, even with shortened waiting times, a number of months may still have elapsed since the patient was entered onto the waiting list. During that time, their medical status may have altered, their specific problem requiring admission may have changed, and the patient's recall of the nature of the procedure, post-procedural regime and potential complications explained to them in the out-patients' clinic may be less than full. All of these issues need to be addressed carefully, and you will play an important part in this process as a Foundation officer.

Aims of the pre-admission clinic include:
- to diagnose the presence of pre-existing medical disease and to make an accurate assessment of the degree of the problem;
- to ensure that the patient is able to receive appropriate information concerning the planned procedure and is able to give informed consent;
- to ensure that the patient's condition is optimized before the procedure, especially if it involves general anaesthesia;
- to ensure that specialized post-procedural care facilities are available if required.

The pre-admission clinic is invariably run by the admitting team, but if there is a general anaesthetic involved, then it should ideally involve an anaesthetist. However, it is unfortunate that in reality, the presence of any anaesthetist at the clinic is an exception rather than the rule.

It may therefore fall to you to assess your patient's fitness for their planned admission. It is the aim of this section is to help you identify the more common problems you will encounter in this situation so that you know how best to deal with them. Remember, difficult problems can always be discussed with anaesthetic and medical colleagues to ensure that the most appropriate management strategy is employed.

Types of admission

There are many situations in which you will be assessing patients and arranging for appropriate investigations and treatment. One of the purposes of your Foundation generic training is to expose you to the wide variety of types of planned admissions.

At the end of your F1 training year you should be happy to prepare and manage patients requiring planned admission in the following scenarios:

- in the Out-patient Clinic;
- in the Pre-admission Clinic;
- at the time of the planned procedure.

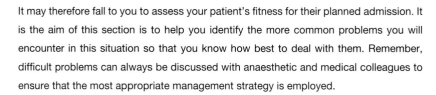

Learning exercise — 1

What specific problems do elderly patients present to the admitting team compared to an otherwise fit, young adult?

See answers to learning exercises on page 99.

Preoperative preparation

Following the admission of a patient for a planned procedure, and before transfer to the operating theatre or other interventional area, several tasks need to be completed to ensure that the patient's procedure and post-procedural management are as successful and efficient as possible.

The following broad categories that might be considered are:

- preparation of the patient;
- checking their preparatory investigations;
- checking their imaging—if any;
- checking the side of the procedure and marking it with a 'permanent' marker;
- checking that the 'list' has been submitted, and/or that it is correct;
- liaising with other health-care professionals as required.

Medication

During your ward routine, you will have observed that many patients are admitted to the hospital on regular medication. Other drugs may be necessary as part of the planned procedure or before and afterwards. Decisions must be made regarding these.

- Is it appropriate for the medication to be continued during the period around the procedure?
- Will regular medications adversely react with necessary medications to be given during the planned admission?
- Will regular medications prejudice the outcome of an anaesthetic, operation or procedure?

▼

- If regular medications are to continue, when should they be stopped before the procedure and recommenced afterwards?
- If the medication is to be stopped, are any alternative medications required?

You should check and be fully conversant with your unit's policies on:

- prophylactic antibiotics;
- perioperative diabetic control;
- management of patients on long-term steroids;
- anaesthetic premedication;
- thromboembolic prophylaxis.

The following exercises will assess your learning needs for preoperative preparation.

Learning exercise 2

a List all the problems that you know to be associated with the drugs listed in Table 1.

b A patient presented with a painful swollen knee following minor trauma, Fig. 1.4.1. Comment on the findings. Which of the drugs listed in Table 1 do you think may have caused this?

Table 1: Pre-admission drugs and associated peri-operative problems

Drug	Problem
Digoxin	
Femodene®	
Warfarin	
Micronor®	
Glyceryl trinitrate	
Cisplatin	
Phenobarbital	
Verapamil	
Alcohol	
Ciprofloxacin	
Lactulose	
Ranitidine	
Chlorphenamine (chlorpheniramine)	
Thyroxine	
Theophylline	
Penicillin	
Gentamicin	
Furosemide (frusemide)	
Aludrox®	
HRT	
Aspirin	
Proton pump inhibitor (e.g. omeprazole)	
Nardil® (monoamine oxidase inhibitor)	
Temazepam	

Drug	Problem
NSAIDs	
Ventolin®	
Prednisolone	
Paracetamol	
Captopril	
Mesalazine	
Chlorpropamide	
Atenolol	

Fig. 1.4.1

Swollen knee following trauma

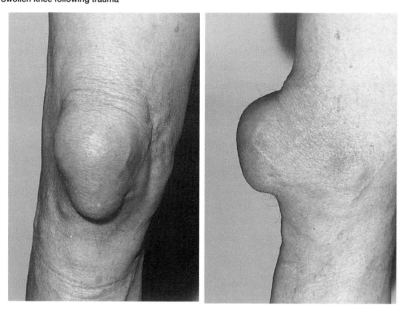

See answers to learning exercises on page 99.

Skin and bowel preparation

Patients themselves have to be optimally prepared to ensure no adverse clinical occurrence. Not so long ago, many patients were visited the day before surgery by the hospital barber for thorough removal of body hair from the operative field. Many patients undergoing abdominal surgery received a full and vigorously uncomfortable 'bowel preparation'. How has this changed in your unit? Review your local policies and work through these learning exercises.

Learning exercise	3

What preoperative skin preparation do patients who are about to undergo surgery require on the ward? What is the rationale and evidence behind the modern policy on skin preparation and hair removal?

Learning exercise	4

In what circumstances might you consider bowel preparation and how?

▼

Answers to learning exercises

1   The main difference between the elderly and the young, fit patient is the existence of co-morbid conditions. Frequently there are social implications too, and if there is likely to be prolonged rehabilitation it is wise to involve the rehabilitation team early in the admission. Elderly patients often become confused in hospital and a prolonged admission may exacerbate this such that they are unable to return home.

2   a   The possible problems associated with the drugs listed are given in Table 2.
     b   The patient had been on long-term warfarin.

Table 2: Pre-admission drugs and associated peri-operative problems

Drug	Problem
Digoxin	Nausea, vomiting, dysrhythmias and heart block (watch K⁺)
Femodene®	Oestrogen-containing contraceptive pill—danger of deep venous thrombosis. Stop 4 weeks before significant surgery
Warfarin	Bleeding. Get international normalized ratio (INR) down to 1.5 before surgery
Micronor®	Progestogen-only pill. No danger
Glyceryl trinitrate	Postural hypotension, tachycardia
Cisplatin	Marrow suppression, ototoxicity, nausea and vomiting: nephrotoxic
Phenobarbital	Cumulative effect with other sedatives, opiates, and hypotensives; nausea and vomiting
Verapamil	Hypotension, bradycardia and heart block
Alcohol	Withdrawal, malnutrition, cardiovascular and liver disease*
Ciprofloxacin	(Allergy: lowers convulsive threshold)
Lactulose	No associated problems
Ranitidine	No associated problems
Chlorphenamine	Cumulative sedative effect with other sedatives
Thyroxine	No particular problems when given in appropriate doses
Theophylline	Vomiting, tachycardia
Penicillin	Allergy (NB cross-reaction with cephalosporin)
Gentamicin	Ototoxicity—care prescribing with renal impairments, monitor levels
Furosemide	?Hypokalaemia: check K⁺ preop especially in elderly patients
Aludrox®	No associated problems
HRT	No associated problems
Aspirin	Bleeding tendency, peptic ulceration, allergy
Proton pump inhibitor (e.g. omeprazole)	Impaired liver function tests (LFTs)
Nardil® (monoamine oxidase inhibitor)	Care with narcotic analgesics, e.g. pethidine
Temazepam	Cumulative effect with other sedatives and analgesics
NSAIDs	Duodenal gastric ulceration and allergy
Ventolin®	Tremor with high dosage
Prednisolone	Defective wound healing, response to sepsis, adrenal suppression
Paracetamol	Care with impaired liver function
Captopril	(Watch renal function), hypotension (especially at start)

Drug	Problem
Mesalazine	Nausea, headache, abdominal pains
Chlorpropamide	Follow proper diabetic control regimens—hypoglycaemia
Atenolol	Bradycardia, cardiac failure, bronchospasm (beware in elderly)

*In addition to the well known effects of alcohol, you should also enquire about other recreational drugs which may affect clinical management.

3   Shaving the day before surgery may cause skin abrasions, which will increase the bacterial count and may encourage sepsis. Thus the operative area is shaved just prior to surgery. Hair traps bacteria and if detached from the skin forms a foreign body and thus needs to be removed from the operative field. At the same time the site for the diathermy pad can also be shaved. There are several types of skin preparation to clean the skin. Iodine and chlorinated hydrocarbons, such as chlorhexidine, may be in an aqueous or alcohol solution. The latter type of solution is flammable and great care needs to be exercised if diathermy is to be used. Alcohol-based solutions should also be avoided in sensitive areas such as the perineum, genitalia or face. Thus the only skin preparation in the ward prior to surgery is to be washed clean with ordinary detergent.

4   Traditionally surgeons have used bowel preparation to remove solid stool prior to operating on the descending and sigmoid colon or rectum. It is not used on the right side as it is not possible to remove the small bowel fluid effluent. A Cochrane Systematic review of randomized controlled studies have not shown any benefit from bowel preparation, thus leaving its routine use in doubt.

For colonoscopy, bowel preparation is clearly imperative to allow proper visualization of the mucosa.

There are special circumstances in upper gastrointestinal surgery where a colonic resection may take place (for example colonic replacement of oesophagus, involvement of colon in gastric or pancreatic cancer) and where bowel preparation is advised.

The common method of bowel preparation consists of a fluid, low-residue diet for several days before surgery and then an oral purgative, such as sodium picosulphate (Picolax®) or polyethyleneglycol solutions, the day before surgery accompanied by intravenous fluids in the elderly.

C ☐
S ☐
R ☐

Preoperative fasting and intravenous fluids

Before surgery and many other procedures, it is necessary for the patient to fast. Why? Again, compare your knowledge of local policies with those discussed in the following learning exercises:

Learning exercise	5
What is a reasonable period of time for a patient to fast before a general anaesthetic?	

Learning exercise	6
What are the dangers of ignoring such advice on 'fasting periods'?	

▼

Learning exercise 7

What special anaesthetic techniques are employed in emergency surgery?

Learning exercise 8

Under what circumstances would you provide intravenous fluids for a patient awaiting surgery? What would be your choice of fluid?

See answers to learning exercises on page 103.

Informed consent

It is likely that obtaining consent from patients will crop up often throughout your career. Traditionally the 'house officer' undertook the task for hospital patients. It is now an accepted practice that any health-care professional consenting a patient must be fully informed about all aspects of the procedure and be competent to answer any questions a patient or their relatives may have. For surgical procedures, the operating surgeon should ideally take the consent. In Unit 3 of this module, you would have studied the moral and legal arguments concerning informed consent in some detail. For now, it is important for you to generally appreciate that good professional practice demands respecting the right of patients to be given enough information about the procedure that you are proposing, so that they can make an informed choice. If you cannot take consent yourself, you should seek a senior colleague to do so, and where appropriate, ask them to train you to take consent.

Check what you already know about consent with these learning exercises.

Learning exercise 9

What topics must be covered in clear, lay language to ensure that you have achieved informed consent for your patient?

Learning exercise 10

List three things that you think will be needed for anticipatory guidance.

See answers to learning exercises on page 103.

Psychological responses

A surgical operation or major interventional procedure is one of life's most frightening experiences. However, while it is a major event in a person's life, to those of us working in a hospital it is an everyday occurrence and we may fail to recognize the profound effect it has on a patient's mental health. Procedures that we might consider minor can be disturbing and even terrifying to the patient, and may evoke significant psychological reactions. It behoves us to understand why the anticipation and experience of surgery has such an intense effect on patients.

It should not be surprising to us that patients have psychological difficulties even if, as medical professionals, we consider these fears to be irrational. Patients are faced with the dangers of the procedure itself, possibly anaesthesia and recovery. To patients, anaesthesia and surgery may be equated with death, mutilation, bizarrely misunderstood anatomical procedures and lasting disability. There is also the overriding fear that an operation always has an exploratory component, and might lead to the discovery of unsuspected, unwanted and terrifying diseases, such as cancer. We have to understand that the resulting depression and anxiety do not 'just happen'. It is our role to identify and understand the significant contributing factors and help our patients understand and cope with them. It should be added that this does not necessarily mean suppressing symptoms by drug treatment as this may be at the expense of understanding what the patient is going through.

We should attempt to anticipate how patients themselves view the experience and then inform, empathize, listen and rehabilitate. We have already learned to do much of this subconsciously and have probably followed the example of our teachers and seniors who are often innately skilled 'psychologists'. Here, however, we will think a little more about the problem of the psychological response to undergoing a major procedure, and dissect your approach to the subject.

Learning exercise   11

What reasons do you think a patient may have for fearing surgery?

See answers to learning exercises on page 103.

You would have learnt more about the importance of communications earlier in Unit 2 of this Module.

Now turn to clinical case 1 to look at a case on cancellation of a planned operation.

Clinical case 1

Mr James Bell is a 74-year-old man with peripheral vascular disease. He is scheduled for a femoropopliteal arterial bypass but on the morning of the operation a patient with a ruptured abdominal aortic aneurysm arrives in the hospital and is operated on in preference to Mr Bell.

Your consultant is busy operating on the emergency and he deputes you to go to the ward and talk to Mr Bell.

Q1 How would you handle the interview with Mr Bell and his relatives explaining to them that the operation has been cancelled?

Clinical case 1 answer

Q1 Patients can understand a cancellation when their own medical condition, for example a chest infection or an abnormal laboratory result, interferes and a benefit can be seen from a temporary delay. In such a case, recognition of the cause of cancellation helps the letdown process. Patients will be disappointed but they will cope.

However, when another patient's needs cause cancellation of an operation, the reaction of the patient whose operation has been cancelled may be quite strong. The patient is psychologically prepared, and may in addition have distressing symptoms, the relief of which would be welcomed, such as the pain of an ischaemic leg in Mr Bell's case. While patients may understand the necessity for emergency procedures to take precedence over their elective operations, it is still a tall order to expect them to consider any case as more important than their own. Careless handling of this situation may precipitate depression, even suicidal tendencies, and serious psychological conflict as patients attempt to balance other people's needs against their own. Such patients inevitably focus on their own problems and fail to empathize with others.

Such patients will feel a sense of outrage at the medical staff and the system but will suppress these feelings because of the realization that their anger is directed at the very people and system upon whom they rely to save their life, relieve their symptoms or correct their problem. Often patients feel that if they have angry thoughts, these will be detected by the medical attendants and that this will be detrimental to their care. So, it is not surprising that patients become depressed. It is remarkably therapeutic if you can bring these feelings into the open. Tell Mr Bell and his relatives that their anger is expected and understandable, that it is safe for them to have these feelings and that it will not jeopardize Mr Bell's relationships with the staff and his treatment. When such a discussion takes place it is usual for any depression to lift immediately.

The approach should be to:

- apologize and explain the facts;
- make a simple statement which shows that you understand the frustration of having an operation cancelled;
- show that you understand the natural human reaction—make a comment which brings the anxieties into the open, such as 'I suppose I would be annoyed and resentful but nobody likes to show their irritation with the surgeons just before they are going to operate on you';
- try to establish before speaking to the patient when the surgery is likely to be rescheduled so that you have some good news for them.

Denial and avoidance: Patients commonly deny or minimize the serious implications of symptoms or an illness. Given the current publicity about cancer, the need for early detection and for periodic check ups, it is remarkable how obviously serious symptoms and signs, such as the presence of a mass or bleeding, are ignored or explained away by otherwise sensible people (including surgeons!). This may be a mechanism for coping in the short term, but it is inappropriate to undermine or challenge these patients. They may be more aware of the truth than we think but in the discussion with patients the choice of words may be vital. Telling a patient that he has a tumour or a malignancy may evoke the response: 'Thank God it isn't cancer!'

Answers to learning exercises

5   The main reason for starving a patient prior to surgery is to ensure an empty stomach at the time of anaesthesia. Traditionally this is usually considered to be 6 hours for food and 2 hours for clear fluids. However opinions on this vary and local practice should be observed. It is important to note that general anaesthesia attenuates the protective laryngeal reflexes and increases the risk of pulmonary aspiration in all kinds of surgical patient. This may further be complicated by delayed gastric emptying

which may occur following trauma, in the critically ill and in those who have sustained head injury or cerebro vascular accident (CVA).

Clearly in life-threatening emergencies, this must be ignored and precautions taken to ensure there is no aspiration of stomach contents in the perioperative period.

6 The danger of not fasting is an increased risk of aspiration of stomach contents.

7 In an emergency, the anaesthetist will use a rapid sequence induction to minimize the risk of aspiration when administering anaesthesia. Techniques used include the use of cricoid pressure (thus ensuring the oesophagus is closed) and intubating the patient with a cuffed tube (preventing aspiration past the tube). A nasogastric tube to empty the stomach may also help. The use of antacid medication will help reduce the complications of aspiration should it occur.

8 Intravenous fluids are required if a patient is likely to be dry or hypovolaemic, or if they are diabetic. The former needs replacement of the lost fluid (for example saline for vomiting and diarrhoea), whereas the latter will require dextrose with a sliding scale of insulin to ensure no hypoglycaemia occurs.

9 To achieve truly informed consent, patients must be given clear information in lay terms about the following:

- The nature of their condition—the diagnosis of the clinical problem to be corrected or managed.
- The proposed treatment—the surgery to be performed to attempt to correct this condition, including the anaesthetic that will be employed.
- The prognosis.
- Recognized side effects of the procedure. For example, these might include the risk of recurrence of the problem of neuralgia, wound infection and other forms of discomfort. The chance of recurrence of the clinical problem should be described.
- Other consequences of the procedure that will affect a patient's day-to-day life—for example the period of bed rest, altered eating patterns and avoidance of particular types of physical activity.
- The special side effects of the problem—for example stomas, specific disfigurement and future disabilities.
- Alternative treatments—including relevant information from the preceding categories—along with the consequences of no treatment.
- Common side effects of the anaesthetic—for example nausea/vomiting, headache, sore throat, post-operative muscular aches.
- Uncommon side effects of the anaesthetic—surgeons should be willing constructively and sensitively to address anxieties about general anaesthesia, including mortality risks.

10 The following would be needed for anticipatory guidance:

- Accurate information. This should include information about the purpose and nature of the proposed operation. There should be an account of the course of events that the patient can expect to occur in the post-operative period. Did you think that the consent guidelines achieved this aim?
- Patients need an opportunity to ask questions and find out what they can do to

cope with events. Often patients will forget to ask these questions at the initial consultation so they should be encouraged to write them down and to refer to them when a later discussion takes place.

- The patient and family members should be given a chance to express their fears and other feelings about the situation, no matter how trivial they may seem to you.
- Patients may minimize the seriousness of the situation and avoid discussion of the operation. This may be a mechanism for coping in the short term and it is not appropriate to undermine or challenge these patients. It is appropriate to follow them up (by whatever mechanism or person) and await the inevitable expression of anxiety, grief or loss (depending on the procedure).

11 Patients may fear surgery for the following reasons:

- Death.
- Primary losses:
  - disability;
  - mutilation.
- Secondary losses:
  - loss of occupation;
  - loss or alteration of roles in society and domestic life;
  - change in personal relationships;
  - change in physical environment, for example changes to the home needed after an amputation or the need to go into residential care;
  - becoming an object of pity or ridicule;
  - being a burden on the family, friends and carers.

There is always a psychological reaction to a physical illness and loss. There may be fear of disablement, for example after amputation of a limb or of mutilation, such as the loss of a breast in mastectomy; and there will be secondary losses such as unemployment, the patient's altered role in society and interference with their personal relationships. Changes in the patient's physical environment are disturbing; these might include a move into a special home or alterations to the patient's own home. Patients also fear that their source of income and security may disappear. People may find themselves the objects of pity or feel stigmatized. Sometimes the loss extends not only to the patient but also to other family members whose lives must change as a result of the patient's illness. Each of these losses must be recognized and faced if patients are to make a satisfactory adjustment to the life that is now open to them.

Other measures

There are other factors and tasks that you must consider in the preoperative preparation of your patient.

You can probably think of many, but do not forget the following:

C ☐
S ☐
R ☐

- Correct site and side marking, for example operative limb/site, stoma position, etc.
- Consideration of a single room if the patient is considered an infectious risk.
- Provision of a neck collar for patients with potential/actual cervical instability, for example rheumatoid patients.

- Use of graduated compression stockings for deep venous thrombosis (DVT) prophylaxis if favoured by your unit.

Checking investigations and images

With the advent of pre-admission clinics, many investigations and images are undertaken prior to the patient's formal admission.

Each team must have a system of checking that the results of investigations and quality of images have been received and checked.

It is dangerous to patients for investigation results to lie unread in hospital computers or ward in-trays. Similarly, in the immediate prelude to admission, images belong on the ward (or are accessible on the PACS system) and not in the Radiology filing rooms.

Optimization

Several factors have been shown to decrease post-operative morbidity and therefore speed up recovery and discharge following surgery. These are often clustered together to optimize patient care. It has been clearly shown that patient education, epidural anaesthesia, transverse incisions and carbohydrate loading can reduce the time to discharge following routine surgery by as much as 50%.

Body mass index

Body mass index (BMI) is a means of allowing for the influence of varying height on body mass. Remember that weight is often confused with mass. Weight is the force exerted by body mass at the gravity level found at normal earth gravity, whereas mass does not vary with gravitational field—a weightless astronaut still has the same body 'mass'. The BMI is widely used in medical research and by the insurance industry for risk prediction, but it is a shorthand trick. Use of the inverse of the square of height equates to body surface area, but some critics have suggested the use of the BMI^3 in which the inverse of the cube of height equates to body volume.

In assessing risk, there are two other factors to be taken into account: body composition and waist circumference. Athletes may have a measured BMI of over 30 kg/m^2, but they have a healthy body composition, with a larger muscle component and little fat. So body composition, especially the proportion of fat mass, is more useful but harder to measure accurately. Moreover males tend to carry excess fat within and around the abdomen, and their waist circumference can be a better guide to risk than their calculated BMI. Normal waist circumferences are <37 inches or 94 cm for men, and < 32 inches or 80 cm for women.

$$BMI = \frac{weight\ (kg)}{(height\ (m))^2}$$

Table 3: Key to BMI

BMI	Classification	Level of health risk
Under 18.5	Underweight	Minimal
18.5–24.9	Normal weight	Minimal
25–29.9	Overweight	Increased
30–34.9	Obese	High
35–39.9	Severely obese	Very high
40–58	Morbidly obese	Extremely high
>60	Super obese risk	Dangerously high

Nutritional assessment

- All surgical patients should have their nutritional state assessed.
- Surgical patients in particular are at great risk of malnutrition and thus subsequent complications.
- Patients can easily be assessed with simple screening tools—your hospital may have a policy on this and it may be part of routine nursing documentation.
- The Malnutrition Universal Screening Tool (MUST), for example, may be used to do this.

Learning exercise	12

Can you describe the American Society of Anaesthesiology's (ASA) system for classifying a patient's general fitness for surgery, and their risk of significant complications including death?

See answers to learning exercises on page 111.

List submission and preoperative liaison

One of the most important events prior to surgery, endoscopy or other interventional procedures is the submission of the 'list'. This may be carried out by your consultant's secretary, by another member of the team or yourself.

For planned procedures, the ordering of the list is likely to be done by the clinician responsible for the list. It is still incumbent upon you to check that the submitted details are correct.

There are likely to be a number of colleagues within the hospital with whom you may have to liaise prior to the list to ensure that there are no delays and everything is prepared as intended.

Learning exercise	13

What details must be present on a submitted operating list?

Learning exercise	14

Which other members of hospital staff might you need to talk to prior to surgery?

See answers to learning exercises on page 111.

Clinical cases 2 and 3 look further at list submission and the need for liaison.

Clinical case 2

The following operating list has been submitted by an orthopaedic team.

Q1 What comments do you have about it?

Q2 What other members of staff would need to be contacted before the list is submitted?

Operating theatre list

Theatre 1: 15 March, 1.30 p.m.

Surgeon(s): Ms Evans and Mr Roberts

Anaesthetist: Dr Campbell

Table 4: Operating list

Order of list	Hospital no.	Surname	First name	DOB	Sex	Ward	Operation
1	245681	Johnson	Walter	63	M	Lister	Debridement of discharging sinus and removal of osteomyelitic bone left 3rd metatarsal head
2	769231	Ruddock	Lily	5/8/25	F	Lister	Revision acetabular cup left hip
3	769231	Jessop	John	2/3/66	M	Lister	Removal of metalwork right tibia
4		Smith	Chris	28/4/66		Day	Removal of ganglion from wrist

Clinical comments:

1 Walter Johnson is an insulin-controlled diabetic. He is colonized with MRSA and has cultured both *Staphylococcus aureus* and *Pseudomonas aeruginosa* from his sinus.

2 Lily Ruddock has rheumatoid arthritis. She is on prednisolone and has an unstable cervical spine.

3 John Jessop is of Afro-Caribbean extraction and has sickle-cell disease.

Clinical case 2 answers

Table 5: Revised operating list

Order of list	Hospital no.	Surname	First name	DOB	Sex	Ward	Operation	Comments
1	428903	Smith	Christine	28/04/66	F	Day	Removal of ganglion from dorsum of left wrist	
2	769231	Ruddock	Lily	5/08/25	F	Lister	Revision acetabular cup left hip.	Charnley hip prosthesis in situ. ?? Requirement for allograft femoral heads Rheumatoid arthritis patient with unstable cervical spine

Order of list	Hospital no.	Surname	First name	DOB	Sex	Ward	Operation	Comments
3	456222	Jessop	John	2/03/66	M	Lister	Removal of i.m. nail right tibia	Russell-Taylor tibial nail with proximal interlocking screws. Image intensifier possibly required. Sickle-cell disease
4	245681	Johnson	Walter	4/02/38	M	Lister	Debridement of discharging sinus and removal of osteomyelitic bone left 3rd metatarsal head	MRSA. Infected case. Diabetic patient

Q1 There are clearly a number of basic mistakes in the list entry:

￢ Missing hospital numbers; duplicated hospital numbers.

￢ Failure to give full date of birth—does 63 refer to age or year of birth?

￢ Failure to give sex of patient who has a first name that could be Christine or Christopher.

￢ There is failure to provide adequate supplementary information concerning the procedures and important medical conditions of the patients.

￢ Finally, there is the question of the list order. This will always be open to debate, but the following guidelines might be adopted for this list:

▼ While it is always desirable for patients such as diabetics and children to go on the front of a list, the presence of an infection overrules this—consequently this case must go last.

▼ The wrist ganglion is a day case. Even if your Day Clinical case Unit remains open until early evening, the patient needs adequate time to recover and consequently should go first at 1.30 p.m.

▼ The list is long for an afternoon and the difficult case is the cup revision. It is difficult to estimate the time of surgery. If it goes second and takes longer than expected, then one has the opportunity to take decisions about the rest of the list, however reluctant you might be to delay any cases.

A suggested revised list is given in Table 5.

Q2 You will need to speak to several people before the list commences:

a Anaesthetist. You will need to speak particularly about:

▼ sickle-cell disease—decisions over anaesthetic and tourniquet;

▼ rheumatoid patient—neck protection and steroid cover;

▼ diabetic patient—diabetic control perioperatively.

b Theatre staff. You will need to speak particularly about:

▼ infected case;

▼ instruments, prosthesis and allograft for the hip revision;

▼ instruments for metalwork removal.

c Microbiology staff. You will need to warn them that specimens will be coming from:

▼ revision hip;

▼ diabetic foot—this may be late coming to the laboratory and will need plating out on arrival.

d Radiographer. Usually removal of metalwork is straightforward, but there are occasions when metalwork can be overgrown, screw heads become stripped and implants fracture. An available image intensifier, if required, is comforting!

Clinical case 3

The following operating list has been submitted by the general surgical team.

Q1 What comments do you have about it?

Q2 What other members of staff would need to be contacted before the list is submitted?

Theatre 7: 12 March, 09.00 a.m.

Surgeon(s): Mr Williams

Anaesthetist: Dr Jones

Table 6: Operating theatre list

Order of list	Hospital no.	Surname	First name	DOB	Sex	Ward	Operation
1	77007	Fraser	David	12/3/94	M	Kids	Inguinal herniotomy
2	63371	Davies	Evan	14/7/23	M	Marks	AP resection rectum
3	55522	Wright	June	23/4/50	F	Marks	Pancreatic resection
4		Macdonald	W	1/2/49	M	Marks	Anal warts

Clinical comment:

1 Mr Macdonald is an HIV-positive haemophiliac.

Clinical case 3 answers

Q1 & 2 Perusal of the submitted list raises the following matters:

a Patient 1 (David Fraser):

▼ No side for inguinal hernia.

▼ Has the patient been marked?

▼ Has the parent been spoken to and consent obtained?

b Patient 2 (Evan Davies):

▼ Has the stoma site been marked?

c Patient 3 (June Wright):

▼ Pancreatic resections frequently need frozen sections.

▼ Has the pathology department been alerted?

d Patient 4 (W. Macdonald):

▼ No unit number.

▼ No first name.

▼ Anaesthetist and theatre staff will need to be informed. Will need to liaise with haematology over factor replacement.

▼ HIV should not be written on list as confidentiality must not be breached.

A suggested revised list is given in Table 7.

Table 7: Revised operating list

Order of list	Hospital no.	Surname	First name	DOB	Sex	Ward	Operation	Comments
1	77007	Fraser	David	12/3/94	M	Kids	Right inguinal herniotomy	
2	63371	Davies	Evan	14/7/23	M	Marks	AP resection rectum	
3	55522	Wright	June	23/4/50	F	Marks	Pancreatic resection	Frozen section arranged
4	77127	Macdonald	William	1/2/49	M	Marks	Anal warts	Haemophilia patient; high-risk patient

Answers to learning exercises

12 Table 8: The ASA system:

Category	Description
I	Fit and healthy patient
II	Mild to moderate systemic disease, which does not cause any functional limitations on the patient
III	Severe systemic disease, which causes functional limitations on a day-to-day basis but is not incapacitating
IV	Severe systemic disease, which presents a significant threat to life
V	Patient is moribund with little expectation of surviving the next 24 h whether managed conservatively or surgically
'E'	The letter E after one of the above grades indicates an emergency procedure

13 The following details must be present on a submitted operating list:

- date and time of surgery;
- surgeon and anaesthetist;
- each patient's full details—name (surname and first name), sex, date of birth, hospital number;
- order of operations;
- full description of operation;
- side to be operated on (if appropriate);
- presence of infection;
- requirement for imaging during surgery.

Some units require additional details, for example diabetes, steroid medication.

14 Prior to surgery there will be liaison with some or all of the following hospital staff members:

- Anaesthetist—ideally, every patient should be discussed with the anaesthetist prior to surgery. You should make sure that the anaesthetist is aware of any medical problem likely to cause concern in the perioperative period. Discuss whether you need to book a bed on the high dependency or intensive care units (critical care level 2 or 3).

- Radiographer—any procedure requiring imaging will require the presence of a radiographer. Make sure they are aware and available to minimize operative delays.
- Pathologist—any specimen taken perioperatively requires correct processing. Some, for example breast biopsies, require immediate examination—the result might influence the course of the rest of the procedure.

Ask the histopathologist in advance if you are in any doubt as to the type, quantity and method of transport required of any biopsy/specimen.

Similarly, many samples taken for microbiological analysis are rendered useless because they are put into an inappropriate medium or left overnight in the operating suite instead of being plated out in the laboratory. If in doubt, speak to the laboratory in advance.

- Physiotherapist/occupational therapist—speak to your physiotherapists and occupational therapists about any special requirements pre- or post-operatively for your patients. Examples might be the establishment of a continuous passive motion machine for a joint in the recovery area following a manipulation or chest physiotherapy prior to operation for patients with cystic fibrosis or bronchiectasis.
- Stoma nurse—the stoma nurse will have wanted to see the patient to discuss stomas and their management, and to help relieve any anxieties. Importantly, they will also mark the best site for ease of care.
- Theatre staff—theatre staff will need to be aware of the following:
- any anticipated difficulties in the planned procedure that may prolong the operating time compared to normal;
- any equipment required that is not normally used for the procedure;
- any implants already in situ, for example the type of metalwork to be removed, design of hip prosthesis to be revised;
- any infection present, for example meticillin-resistant *Staphylococcus aureus* (MRSA) (formerly methicillin-resistant *Staphylococcus aureus*), HIV, contaminated wounds;
- Ward staff—ward staff need to be given as much information as possible about the procedure and post-operative regime, especially when the procedure is unusual.
- Other medical teams involved in the patient's care—prior to surgery, inform any in the immediate care of the patient around the time of the procedure, for example oncologists, radiotherapists, nutrition team.
- Other surgical teams—during out-of-hours periods, when shared emergency lists are commonplace in most hospitals, it is important that common professional respect and courtesies are maintained when booking cases. At times, there may be disagreement between surgical teams on the relative priorities of patients. Direct conversation and an awareness of the concerns of other teams should lead to an amicable resolution of any impasse.
- Inform Intensive Care or HDU staff to arrange a bed for high risk surgical patients.

C ☐
S ☐
R ☐

Pre-admission investigations

- Preoperative investigations should be planned with respect to the patients ASA status and grade of surgery (minor, intermediate or major).

  NICE now publish guidelines about which tests should be used: www.nice.org.uk

You will find that your assessment of any patient will make more sense if you always have in mind the association between:

- anaemia,
- respiratory function, and
- cardiac function.

It is worthwhile at this point spending a little time on understanding what this association means.

The most important function of these systems is the supply of oxygen (and nutrients) to the cells of the body. The oxygen flux equation is the product of:

Cardiac output × **Arterial saturation** × **Respiratory function** × **Haemoglobin (Hb)**

and this measures the amount of oxygen that is delivered in 1 min.

We know that 1 g of Hb when fully saturated will combine with 1.39 ml of oxygen. Therefore the oxygen flux equation is as follows:

$5000 × 95\% × 15\% × 1.39 = 990 \sim 1000$ ml/min

Assumes:

- Cardiac output = 5000 ml/min
- Arterial saturation = 95%
- Respiratory function = 15 g/100 ml

As you can see from this, in a healthy individual, 1000 ml of oxygen is delivered to the various tissues every minute. Of this amount, only about 250 ml is utilized by the conscious resting subject—the **basal metabolic rate** (BMR).

Arterial blood therefore loses 25% (250 ml) of its oxygen content, and the blood returning to the heart (the mixed venous blood) is approximately 75% saturated. This 75% saturated blood (containing 750 ml O_2) forms an important reserve which may be drawn on under various forms of stress.

The Hb molecule, when fully saturated, combines with four molecules of O_2. It is therefore convenient to consider that during every circulation, each Hb molecule need release only one of its four molecules of combined O_2 to satisfy the BMR, and the Hb in mixed venous blood is combined with three out of the possible four:

$Hb(O_2)_4 \longrightarrow Hb(O_2)_3$

100%   75% saturated
saturated   venous blood (oxygen reserve)
arterial blood

Because of the complexities of the very large Hb molecule, it has different affinities for oxygen depending on how saturated it is. It is relatively easy to remove the first oxygen molecule, as above, but progressively more difficult to remove the others, as the Hb molecule has a greater affinity for oxygen the less it has.

Therefore, in theory, if arterial blood were only 75% saturated, it would still deliver 750 ml O_2/min, and easily satisfy the oxygen flux equation by delivering much more than the 250 ml required for the BMR. However, in practice it is much more difficult for the various tissues to extract the oxygen that is required because the Hb molecule tries harder to hold on to its diminished amount. In other words, it is **delivered**, but is not necessarily readily **available**. Despite the varying numbers of the oxygen flux equation, it is important to always remember:

The more saturated the blood, the better the patient.

Although the oxygen flux equation must always be satisfied, it is important to note that it is the **product** of **three variables**. It is for this reason that any one abnormality (in either Hb, heart or lung function) is assessed, not as an isolated problem, but with regard to its association with the other two variables.

If one variable is halved (for example cardiac output) and the other two variables (lung function and Hb) are unchanged, then the oxygen flux is halved (500 ml/min). This is obviously not good, but nevertheless, more oxygen will be delivered than is actually required for the BMR. However, that leaves very little in reserve; delivery does not necessarily equate to availability.

If any two variables are halved (for example cardiac output and Hb) then the oxygen flux is reduced to a quarter (250 ml/min). This is a very dangerous situation. The BMR can barely be met, and there is no reserve at all.

If all three variables are halved, the oxygen flux is reduced to one-eighth, or 125 ml of O_2/min. This value is below the BMR, and if maintained for any length of time is incompatible with life. Hence, although the reduction in each individual variable is not in itself lethal, in combination such reductions can be.

These quantitative implications of the oxygen flux have been extensively explored, and the conclusion to be stressed is that: the criteria for the adequacy of each variable can only be considered in relation to the other variables. The example given above, of progressively halving each variable, is an extreme case. In reality we are commonly faced with smaller variations of this. Thus, a degree of arterial hypoxaemia, which may be tolerated in an otherwise healthy patient, may be dangerous in patients with impaired cardiac output or anaemia.

The three variables may be conveniently displayed as in Fig. 1.4.2, which clearly shows the possibilities of the combinations of any two variables or even all three together.

Fig. 1.4.2

Venn diagram to show oxygen flux equation variables: haemoglobin, cardiac output and arterial saturation (lung function).

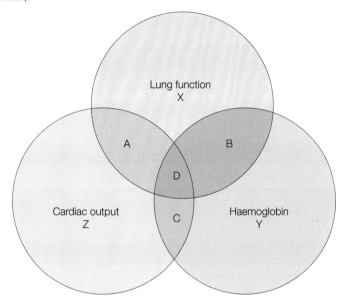

For example, the combination of anaemia and low cardiac output, which occurs in untreated haemorrhage, is shown in Area C. If the patient also then suffered from acute respiratory distress syndrome (ARDS), the patient would move into real danger zone D.

On a more cheerful note, it is helpful that all patients have homeostatic mechanisms, all of which are designed to drag the oxygen flux equation back towards normal. So in chronic conditions compensations are more normal.

A patient with a low arterial saturation, due perhaps to chronic obstructive pulmonary disease (COPD), chronic smoking, or living at altitude, would be represented in Area X. Homeostatic mechanisms would try to compensate and return the oxygen flux by:

- providing a high Hb level (secondary polycythaemia);
- increasing heart rate and cardiac output.

Similarly a patient with a low Hb, due to a chronic bleed, dietary anaemia, chronic renal failure, etc. (Area Y), would be compensated by an increase in cardiac output. (In this instance the lung function cannot be increased beyond the 100% saturation.)

Such examples provide a classic example of the importance of viewing the patient as a whole.

The question of the lowest Hb concentration permissible for major surgery can only be answered after consideration of:

- the actual and projected cardiac output before, during and after surgery;
- pulmonary function during and after surgery.

As an introduction to the influence of coexisting diseases on the preparation of a patient for surgery, try the following learning exercises.

▼

> **Learning exercise**   15
>
> List six relevant points that you would look for in the physical examination of a patient with known pulmonary disease.

> **Learning exercise**   16
>
> When you take a history from an elderly patient suspected of having a cardiac problem, list five questions you would ask them in the out-patients clinic and give the reason for each.

> **Learning exercise**   17
>
> Suppose that a patient with impaired cardiac function was to undergo a major aortic reconstruction. What subjective and objective assessment of cardiac performance can be made before, during or after the operation?

> **Learning exercise**   18
>
> What aspects of renal function can be measured fairly simply, in someone with renal failure?

Heart disease

While reading the text try to clarify in your mind the most common cardiac conditions you are likely to encounter in the preoperative work-up of your patients, how they may best be managed and how you can influence their progress perioperatively. A careful history and examination will go a long way towards diagnosing the more common cardiac problems that will affect the patient's perioperative course. Remember that in the pre-assessment clinic, this is equally if not more important than assessment of the surgical condition involved. This point is often overlooked—there is no point in scheduling a case if the patient is likely to die as a result of the surgery!

Approximately half of the life-threatening complications that occur perioperatively are cardiac, in particular:

- myocardial ischaemia;
- myocardial infarction (MI);
- congestive cardiac failure;
- dysrhythmias.

Recent years have seen continuing improvements in anaesthesia and regional blocks have become increasingly popular again. However, it must be stressed that in patients undergoing non-cardiac surgery, there is no proven difference in short- or long-term cardiac morbidity between central nerve block (epidural/spinal) and general anaesthesia.

However, there are many benefits that the patient might experience with regional or local anaesthesia, in particular better post-operative pain relief. This will improve oxygenation with better respiratory function, and reduce the need for opiates, which might lead to respiratory depression and hypoxia.

In STEP™ Foundation Module 3 you will look in more detail at cardiac anatomy and physiology. This will include close interpretation of electrocardiograms (ECGs) and cardiac arrhythmias.

Aims of pre-admission assessment include:

- detection of cardiovascular disease;
- assessment of severity of disease;
- assessment of the functional reserve;
- consideration of likely benefits of surgery balanced against risks;
- preoperative optimization of the patient, by either medical or surgical treatment;
- minimization of perioperative complications.

Strategies for assessing fitness for surgery include:

- establishing whether cardiac condition is stable or unstable;
- establishing whether medical management will improve condition;
- how the condition is likely to affect perioperative course?

Learning exercise	19

Write out the clinical features of importance, the risks, and the preoperative and operative measures to be considered for patients presenting with the following cardiac conditions:

a   mitral stenosis

b   atrial fibrillation

c   heart block

d   aortic stenosis?

Answers to learning exercises

General considerations

15   Six points in the physical examination of a patient with pulmonary disease are:

1   barrel-shaped chest;

2   using the accessory muscles of respiration;

3   pursing the lips/dyspnoea at rest;

4   clubbing of fingers;

5   colour of sputum;

6   cyanosis.

16   Five questions to ask a patient with suspected cardiac disease are listed in Table 9.

Table 9: Questions to ask when examining a patient with suspected cardiac disease

Question	Reason
Do you have any chest pain and, if so, what brings it on?	Is it angina?
Do you get shortness of breath on lying down, or any ankle swelling?	Is there congestive heart failure?
Does your heart ever race or miss beats?	Is there intermittent or persistent dysrhythmia?
Have you ever had a MI or high BP?	Is this a risk factor and what is the severity of ischaemia?
Do you smoke?	Is this a further risk factor? Should be stopped prior to operation

17 Cardiac performance should be assessed prior to surgery by the following tests (NB: not all patients need all these tests):

- A history may elicit some of the symptoms, as illustrated above. This gives a rough estimate of risk.
- Clinical examination: for example raised jugular venous pressure, triple rhythm dysrhythmias, ankle swelling, lung crepitations, exercise tolerance.
- ECG and cardiac enzymes.
- Exercise test (with ECG).
- Ejection fraction of the left ventricle as measured by colour duplex Doppler ultrasound. A level of 40% is a crude 'cut-off' value.
- Coronary angiography.

(NB: The latter four investigations can be used to defer major surgery in otherwise unsuspected at-risk patients.)

- Cardiac output. This can be measured by a thermal dilution method employing a Swan–Ganz catheter. This instrument can also estimate a series of intracardiac pressures, particularly pulmonary wedge pressure (left atrial pressure), which is a reflection of left ventricular function. Less invasive measures such as Lithium dilution can now be used.
- Thallium scan.

18 Some simple methods of measuring renal function include:

- Urine volume. The usual minimum urinary volume is approximately 0.5 ml/kg/h, and anything much less than this, for example 20 ml/h, is oliguric.
- Specific gravity of the urine, and urinalysis to search for protein or blood (dipstix) and to see if the kidney is able to concentrate the urine. Water loading and deprivation tests would further elucidate this.
- Serum creatinine and blood urea levels. Creatinine levels are a more sensitive way of looking at impairment of renal function. Creatinine clearance levels will form a useful baseline on which to assess or follow overall renal function.
- MSU (mid-stream specimen or urine) or CSU (catheter specimen of urine) to indicate the presence or absence of urinary tract infection (UTI), and urine microscopy to look for casts and cells.
- The measurement of urinary electrolytes (coupled with serum electrolyte levels) may indicate the ability of the kidney to retain or lose significant amounts of sodium or potassium.
- Osmolality. This is a reflection of the total solute concentration of the solution. Osmolality should be even throughout all body compartments, i.e. about 290 mosmol/kg. The kidneys can increase osmolality fourfold when there is severe fluid deficit. With fluid deprivation (8 h) the urine: plasma ratio should be >2.

Heart disease

19 The chief clinical features, associated risks and precautionary measures for mitral stenosis, atrial fibrillation and heart block are shown in Table 10:

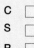

C ☐
S ☐
R ☐

Table 10: Clinical features, associated risks and precautionary measures for mitral stenosis, atrial fibrillation and heart block

	Clinical features	Risks	Perioperative precautions
(a) Mitral stenosis	Mitral facies Diastolic murmur Look for AF and/or RVF Is patient taking anticoagulants?	Few, if mild or moderate Endocarditis Fluid overload	ECG, CXR, serum K⁺ if on diuretics, and INR if on anticoagulants Prophylactic antibiotics Avoid swings in blood pressure Cautious transfusion and fluid balance
(b) Atrial fibrillation	Pulse and ECG Determine cause, e.g. IHD, thyroxicosis, valvular heart disease, sepsis, arterial embolism (if not on anticoagulants) Ca bronchus	Cardiac decompensation and failure Arterial embolism (if not on anticoagulants)	Treat cause Check digoxin level If surgery is urgent, control with digoxin or amiodarone. Monitor Avoid HR rises. May need higher filling pressures. Atropine to restore AV conduction
(c) Heart block	ECG will determine 1st-degree, or complete block Is it due to Digoxin effect?	Severe bradycardia or cardiac arrest	Atropine to restore AV conduction Check digoxin level ?Prophylactic pacing with major surgery and second-degree block, and always with third-degree block Avoid verapamil, β-adrenergic antagonists Have atropine, isoprenaline and the means for temporary pacing to hand
(d) Aortic stenosis	Angina Drop attacks Exhaustion	Perioperative cardiovascular collapse	Echocardiogram to assess severity of stenosis Cardiological opinion Postpone non-urgent surgery pending expert review

Ischaemic heart disease

In an ischaemic heart disease (IHD), the basis of management stems from the fact that myocardial ischaemia will occur whenever the balance between myocardial oxygen supply and demand is disturbed such that demand exceeds supply.

Major determinations of myocardial oxygen supply

The following are used to determine myocardial oxygen supply:

- Coronary perfusion pressure—aortic diastolic pressure minus left ventricular end-diastolic pressure.
- Diastolic time.

Major determinations of myocardial oxygen demand

The following factors influence myocardial oxygen demand:

- heart rate;
- inotropic state;
- afterload (impedance to the left ventricular ejection);
- preload (left ventricular end-diastolic pressure—the 'filling' pressure).

Factors that decrease supply or increase demand must be avoided in the perioperative period. An increase in heart rate may be detrimental as it increases oxygen demand while at the same time decreasing supply—a recipe for disaster. A significant decrease in systemic arterial pressure (diastolic pressure drop of 20% or more of normal) must not be allowed to occur as this will decrease coronary perfusion. While not necessarily a problem in the normal heart, an area of critical stenosis will be severely tested.

So much for the theory. How does this affect your clinical practice? Well, the areas you should concentrate on will include:

- Good attention to post-operative analgesia as pain will lead to hypertension and tachycardia (increasing the demand for oxygen).
- Close attention to appropriate fluid therapy as hypovolaemia will reduce oxygen supply (reduced blood pressure [BP]).

Prompt management of arrhythmias

Supplementary oxygen is important to maximize delivery of oxygen to the tissues. If the BP falls or delivery is compromised for whatever reasons, maximizing the oxygen saturation will help to ensure adequate delivery under periods of stress. It is customary to give oxygen supplements continuously for the first 24 hours and then overnight for the next three nights. Prescribe this on the drug chart to ensure it is given by the ward staff. Myocardial ischaemia is known to occur during these nights in many patients.

Learning exercise	20

Assume you are in the pre-admission clinic and assessing a patient for a hernia repair who has coexisting cardiac problems. What are the aims of perioperative management of this patient?

Learning exercise	21

How may IHD present to you preoperatively?

Learning exercise	22

A 65-year-old diabetic male patient with mild hypertension presents for a hernia repair. He has no symptoms of angina at rest or on exercise. Can we assume that he presents no risk as far as coronary artery disease is concerned?

See answers to learning exercises on page 125.

It goes without saying that once you have established the presence of cardiac disease you must perform a thorough history and examination. It is worth noting that what we are trying to establish is the functional behaviour and reserve of the heart, that is, what it can do under stress. This will help us to assess how it will behave when undergoing the various rigours of the perioperative period. You should try to consider how best to achieve this.

Having taken a careful medical history and performed an examination to establish the presence and severity of cardiac disease, what investigations are at your disposal to assist you in your assessment?

Again, the important issue here is the functionality of the heart, i.e. what happens when the heart is made to work. A number of investigations may be normal when the heart is rested but show significant changes when stressed. Many of the manoeuvres the anaesthetist performs result in a potential stress to the heart (for example intubation, extubation), and surgical pain can cause significant tachycardia and hypertension. These

▼

situations stress the heart and may cause ischaemia in the diseased heart.

Some points to note regarding the investigations are as follows:

- The resting ECG may be normal in patients with significant coronary artery disease (at least 30% of patients presenting for vascular surgery who had a normal ECG have significant coronary artery disease).
- Exercise ECG will correlate better with perioperative complications if it shows ischaemic episodes or the patient is unable to reach 85% of maximum heart rate.
- Echocardiography does not assess the coronaries but gives an idea of global cardiac function and valve disease. It has become essential in the assessment of murmurs detected in the perioperative period.
- Stress echocardiography and thallium scanning are more sophisticated investigations to show up areas of ischaemia.
- Coronary angiography provides the definitive evidence of coronary occlusion.

Assessment of severity

As we have seen, the crucial aspect of assessing cardiac disease perioperatively is the ability of the myocardium to withstand the various stresses imposed on it by the operation and anaesthesia. At rest the patient may exhibit few symptoms because the myocardium is easily able to cope with the workload imposed upon it. However, on exercise it may struggle, resulting in symptoms and signs of myocardial insufficiency— namely angina, shortness of breath, etc. It is this assessment of myocardial reserve that best predicts the ability of the heart to cope with the rate, pressure and oxygen changes which it might encounter. Most of the above investigations are elaborate and expensive, but what we need in the pre-admission clinic is an easy and reliable method for assessing the severity of the patient's cardiac disease.

Most of the classification systems utilize this functionality to grade the severity of IHD. The two most common are in Tables 11 and 12:

Table 11: Classification of patients with heart disease (New York Heart Association)

Class	Description
1	Asymptomatic
2	Symptoms with ordinary activity, but comfortable at rest
3	Symptoms with minimal activity, but comfortable at rest
4	Symptoms at rest

Table 12: Risk of perioperative MI (New York Heart Association)

Class	Description
1	Angina with strenuous exercise
2	Angina with moderate exercise
3	Angina after climbing one flight of stairs
4	Angina with any exercise

Patients in classes 1 and 2 in the Table 12 are at no increased risk from surgery, but should have an exercise ECG prior to surgery. Anti-angina therapy should be continued throughout the perioperative period. Patients in classes 3 and 4 should be considered for coronary angiography and possibly coronary artery surgery prior to major elective surgery, because of the high incidence of MI when elective surgery is undertaken on this group. If you are confronted with a patient who fits into this group you should seek a cardiology opinion regarding further investigation and cardiac management.

Strategies for risk reduction

Once the level of risk is identified, there are a variety of strategies which may be put into place to reduce cardiac risk:

- Alter risk factors:
  - optimize medical treatment while postponing surgery if possible;
  - perform less invasive or shorter procedure;
  - abandon surgery altogether.
- Alter perioperative care:
  - involve only senior anaesthetists and surgeons;
  - Institute early invasive cardiovascular monitoring;
  - preoperative optimization on intensive care unit (ICU) or HDU;
  - post-operative care on ICU or HDU;
  - elective post-operative ventilation.
- Meticulous attention to detail:
  - adequate analgesia;
  - treat arrhythmias;
  - supplemental oxygen for prolonged periods;
  - continuation of patient's normal drug regime;
  - check Hb.

Learning exercise	23

What are the main symptoms that you will look for when assessing a patient with cardiac disease?

Learning exercise	24

In the same patient what signs would you try to elicit in your examination?

Learning exercise	25

What simple investigations could you do to help in your preoperative assessment?

Learning exercise	26

What particular aspects of these symptoms and signs would you use to estimate the risk for that patient undergoing surgery?

See answers to learning exercises on page 125.

Now work through clinical case 4, which guides you through the preoperative assessment of such a patient.

Clinical case 4

Mr Jones has osteoarthritis of his knee, and this requires replacing. He attends your routine Pre-admission Checking Clinic today, which is 3 weeks before his scheduled operation. He smokes 20 cigarettes a day, but denies any shortness of breath.

He was well until 4 months ago, when, while on holiday, he was admitted to Coronary Care in another hospital with severe chest pain. A letter from that hospital states that he did in fact have a MI, confirmed by raised cardiac enzymes. ECG changes are consistent with an antero-lateral infarct.

He now takes the following: low-dose aspirin; atenolol; enalapril; simvastatin; sublingual glyceryltrinitrate (GTN) p.r.n. (on average 1–2 times/day).

Q1   How would you assess the severity of Mr Jones' symptoms?

Q2   Why is the assessment of angina important?

Q3   How would you manage his admission in 3 weeks' time?

Q4   What advice would you give the patient?

Q5   What else might you do?

Mr Jones is in fact assessed by the anaesthetist that same day, and understands the need for a delay to his treatment. He goes home to await a letter to attend the cardiologist's out-patient clinic. Unfortunately he is admitted to your casualty department a week later, with right iliac fossa pain, pyrexia and vomiting. He is diagnosed as having an acute appendicitis, requiring operation. In the meantime you have finished your F1 orthopaedic post and are now the F1 General Surgical officer on call, when you meet up with Mr Jones again.

Q6   What are your strategies for risk reduction?

Q7   What is the goal of management of the ischaemic myocardium?

Q8   How can delivery of oxygen to the myocardium be maximized?

Q9   Why is perioperative analgesia important in the management of myocardial ischaemia?

Q10   How else can myocardial oxygen consumption be reduced?

Clinical case 4 answers

Q1   The severity of Mr Jones' symptoms is assessed as follows:
  ¬ Pain/dyspnoea at rest.
  ¬ Orthopnoea/paroxysmal nocturnal dyspnoea in cardiac failure.
  ¬ ECG—probably will only confirm presence of MI.
  ¬ Exercise tolerance test—you will see that he probably sits somewhere between class 2 and 3 (see Table 12). This assesses the functionality of his heart.
  ¬ Echocardiography, preoperatively to assess left ventricular function.

Q2   All patients with IHD are high risk. In addition, angina post-infarct is ominous as it suggests a continued area of threatened myocardium. If he has an infarction

▼

perioperatively, this will carry a 40%–60% mortality rate. In addition, it might be possible to optimize his medical treatment prior to surgery, thereby reducing his risk.

Q3 You would manage his planned admission in 3 weeks quite simply—cancel the operation!

The risk of perioperative MI is most strongly correlated with previous infarction history, or the presence of inadequately treated cardiac failure. Prior MI carries an increased rate of reinfarction:

- MI <3 months ago = 30%–35%
- MI 3–6 months ago = 10%–15%
- MI >6 months ago = 6%
- No previous MI = 0%–5%

This operation MUST be delayed until at least 6 months after his MI, to minimize his risk factors.

Q4 You would advise Mr Jones to stop smoking!

Q5 Other steps you could take would be to alert the anaesthetist and the cardiologist, so that they may together follow his preop progress and decide upon the optimum time to operate, and advise you of this.

Q6 In general, the high-risk patient should undergo the quickest possible procedure during daylight hours with a surgeon and anaesthetist of sufficient seniority to minimize the risks of early surgical and anaesthetic complications. Mr Jones, now only 4 months post-MI, is in the high-risk group. Any cardiac medication should be continued throughout the operative period. He may benefit from invasive cardiac monitoring and admission to ITU post-operatively.

Q7 The principal goal in managing the ischaemic myocardium is to ensure its adequate oxygenation by:
- increasing the available oxygen to the myocardium;
- minimizing oxygen consumption by the myocardium.

Q8 Oxygen delivery to the myocardium is maximized as follows:
- Give supplementary oxygen. Oxygen should be given for the first 24 h, and then overnight for at least the next 3 nights. Prescribe this on the drug chart.
- Avoid marked anaemia; keep Hb >10 (remember the oxygen flux equation).
- Ensure adequate diastolic pressure, and keep the heart rate low to ensure a long diastolic time to help maintain a good coronary flow. Remember that the myocardium is only perfused during diastole. A tachycardia will therefore reduce myocardial oxygenation by increasing oxygen consumption and reducing delivery.

Q9 Perioperative analgesia is important because a patient in pain will mount a tachycardia and will raise their BP. Such an increase in both chronotropy and inotropy will markedly increase the myocardial oxygen consumption, increasing the risk of an ischaemic or infarctive event. It is very important therefore that good post-operative analgesia is maintained over the first post-operative week.

Q10 Myocardial oxygen consumption can also be reduced by avoiding hypothermia or hyperthermia. Hypothermia will cause shivering, leading to an increase in general oxygen consumption/demand, while hyperthermia will cause a tachycardia, increasing myocardial oxygen demand and reducing its supply during a shortened diastole. Afterload can be reduced with vasodilators. The work of breathing may be reduced by the use of elective ventilation.

Answers to learning exercises

Ischaemic heart disease

20 The aims of perioperative management include:

- detection of cardiovascular disease;
- assessment of severity of disease;
- assessment of the functional reserve;
- consideration of likely benefits of surgery balanced against risks;
- preoperative optimization of the patient either by medical or surgical treatment;
- minimization of perioperative complications.

21 Possible presenting features of IHD include:

- angina—stable or unstable;
- cardiac failure;
- arrhythmia;
- previous MI;
- silent disease.

22 This patient cannot be assumed to present no risk of coronary artery disease. Of episodes of myocardial ischaemia, 75% may be silent. In view of his risk factors (age, diabetes, hypertension) he should be treated as if he has coronary artery disease.

23 When assessing a patient with cardiac disease, the main symptoms to look for include:

- angina;
- previous MI;
- shortness of breath;
- peripheral vascular disease;
- arrhythmia.

24 The signs to look for in a patient with cardiac disease should include:

- raised jugular venous pressure;
- enlarged left ventricle;
- basal crepitations;
- added sounds;
- ankle swelling.

25 ECG and chest X-ray are the basic investigations for preoperative assessment of a patient with cardiac disease. If you are more worried, then an echo can establish the overall state of the myocardium. Once you are getting into the realms of stress testing and angiography you should probably be consulting with a cardiologist.

C ☐
S ☐
R ☐

26   With regard to the history, the following factors are used in estimating the risks of surgery for a patient with cardiac disease:

- exercise tolerance and limiting factors;
- NYHA functional class;
- MI within 6 months;
- paroxysmal nocturnal dyspnoea (PND);
- orthopnoea;
- type of surgery.

Hypertension

Pre-admission assessment

When assessing a patient who is found to have raised blood pressure, the history, examination and investigations should be targeted at establishing evidence of end-organ damage and associated cardiovascular pathology, for example:

- left ventricular hypertrophy;
- myocardial ischaemia;
- congestive cardiac failure;
- aortic aneurysms;
- renal impairment;
- cerebral haemorrhages;
- retinal changes.

It is also necessary to rule out possible secondary causes as listed below.

Assessment of end-organ damage and associated cardiovascular pathology will help to decide two things:

1 whether the hypertension is long-standing or simply a one-off reading in a nervous patient in a threatening situation;
2 what mode of treatment is best suited for a particular patient.

Learning exercise	27

What do you know to be major risks to hypertensive patients in the perioperative period?

Learning exercise	28

a What symptoms would help you ascertain evidence of end-organ disease associated with the hypertension?
b What might you find on examination?
c What investigations would further support your diagnosis?

See answers to learning exercises on page 130.

The vast majority of cases of hypertension are idiopathic ('essential') and respond to therapy. Recent onset and refractory hypertension should prompt a search for secondary causes as these may require specific treatment.

Secondary causes of hypertension

Suspicion of secondary hypertension will require further investigation, such as renal ultrasound or echocardiography.

- Renal:
  - chronic glomerulonephritis; chronic atrophic pyelonephritis;
  - congenital polycystic kidneys;
  - renal artery stenosis.
- Endocrine:
  - Conn's syndrome;
  - adrenal hyperplasia;
  - phaeochromocytoma;
  - Cushing's syndrome;
  - acromegaly.
- Cardiovascular:
  - coarctation of aorta.
- Pregnancy.
- Drugs.

It is particularly important to rule out or confirm phaeochromocytoma as a cause because of high intra-operative morbidity and mortality in surgery on patients with this undiagnosed tumour.

Clinical management

Once you have detected hypertension and established that it is chronic and not 'white-coat' induced, what are your management options?

- If mild or moderate hypertension (diastolic <110 mmHg) is found and there is no evidence of metabolic or cardiovascular abnormalities, there is no need to delay surgery, though a beta-adrenergic blocker, for example atenolol, given as a premedication, has been shown to reduce perioperative myocardial ischaemia.
- Treated hypertensives should take their routine medication on the day of surgery, particularly if they take beta-blockers or clonidine, as abrupt cessation of these drugs can cause rebound hypertension and tachycardia.
- If hypertension is severe (diastolic >110 mmHg), elective surgery should be delayed to allow appropriate and effective management. This should be done by the patient's own GP or with the help of the physicians. It is advisable to have at least 1 month of treatment before reconsidering surgery.

Learning exercise	29

Why is it so important to control hypertension prior to surgery?

Learning exercise	30

What morbidity might the patient encounter perioperatively if surgery is continued in the face of uncontrolled hypertension?

▼

Learning exercise	31

What lines of treatment are available to control the hypertension?

Learning exercise	32

Once the hypertension is controlled what increased risk does the patient possess?

Learning exercise	33

If you do admit a patient with poorly controlled hypertension, and urgent surgery is mandatory, what steps can be taken?

See answers to learning exercises on page 130.

Clinical case 5

James Simpson, 56 years old, presents on the ward 24 h before an elective inguinal hernia repair. He is asymptomatic but on examination is noted to have a BP of 170/100 mmHg. No other abnormal signs are identified on examination.

Q1 Is this BP abnormal?

You decide to admit him anyway and prepare him for theatre.

Q2 What investigations does this patient need?

Q3 Should surgery be delayed until after any treatment?

Clinical case 5 answers

Q1 The BP is slightly high. However, this may be what used to be referred to as 'white-coat' hypertension. A single elevated non-invasive BP does not indicate chronic hypertension, though it may indicate increased likelihood of intra-operative hypertension and associated complications.

Q2 All patients, irrespective of age, having elevated preop hypertension require:
   ⊓ urea, creatinine and electrolytes—for diagnosing renal impairment;
   ⊓ ECG—for looking for left ventricular hypertrophy, ischaemia, conduction defects;
   ⊓ Chest X-ray—for identifying cardiomegaly or pulmonary oedema.

Q3 There is no evidence that if mild to moderate essential hypertension (diastolic <110 mmHg) with no end-organ damage or associated cardiovascular pathology is found in the preoperative assessment of elective surgical patients there is benefit in delaying surgery. Ordinarily, once the patient has got used to his surroundings blood pressure frequently settles. He may benefit from a sedative premed.

If severe hypertension (diastolic >110 mmHg) is found and continues while admitted, in the elective patient, there is proven benefit in delaying surgery and adequately treating the BP over the course of at least 1 month.

Clinical case 6

56-year-old Daniel Lee presents 24 h before his elective inguinal hernia repair. He gives a history of paroxysmal episodes of anxiety, flushing, palpitations, headaches and tremor. His BP readings vary, one noted to be as high as 230/120 mmHg and another one 140/90 mmHg. There are no other abnormal signs.

Q1 What is a possible diagnosis?

Q2 Are there any further investigations that may be useful?

Q3 What is the further management of this patient?

Q4 a What are the other causes of secondary hypertension
   b What are the complications of hypertension?

Clinical case 6 answers

Q1 These symptoms and signs may be caused by a phaeochromocytoma. If hypertension is found in the previously normal preoperative patient, then history and examination should be directed to eliciting possible causes of secondary hypertension, and in eliciting end-organ damage and cardiovascular complications.

Q2 Further investigations in this instance are urinary vanillylmandelic acid (VMA), CT/ MRI of abdomen, etc. Again, special investigations directed towards possible causes or sequelae of hypertension will be suggested by the history and examination.

Q3 Often when a secondary cause of hypertension is suspected, surgery can be justifiably delayed to warrant further investigation and treatment. Phaeochromocytoma particularly should be excluded as this can cause life-threatening complications, the chances of which can be reduced with appropriate preoperative treatment.

Q4 a Other secondary causes of hypertension include:
   ▾ Renal-chronic glomerulonephritis; chronic atrophic pyelonephritis; congenital polycystic kidneys; renal artery stenosis.
   ▾ Endocrine—Conn's syndrome; adrenal hyperplasia; phaeochromocytoma; Cushing's syndrome; acromegaly.
   ▾ Cardiovascular—coarctation of the aorta.
   ▾ Pregnancy
   ▾ Drugs.
   b Complications of chronic hypertension include:
   ▾ Left ventricular hypertrophy
   ▾ Myocardial ischaemia
   ▾ Congestive cardiac failure
   ▾ Aortic aneurysms
   ▾ Renal impairment
   ▾ Cerebral haemorrhages
   ▾ Retinal changes

Answers to learning exercises

Hypertension

27 Hypertension (BP >160/95 mmHg) is a common condition and a risk factor for peripheral and cerebral vascular disease and coronary artery disease. Studies have shown that although hypertension is not an independent risk factor for perioperative cardiovascular complications, it is associated with intra-operative BP fluctuations (particularly hypotension) and myocardial ischaemia, which can in themselves cause significant perioperative morbidity and mortality. These fluctuations can be prevented by appropriate preoperative treatment. Intra-operative myocardial ischaemia correlates with post-operative cardiac morbidity, and prolonged intra-operative hypotension also increases the risk of post-operative cardiac and renal complications.

28 a Symptoms of significant end-organ damage due to hypertension might include:
      • angina (exertional chest pain);
      • cardiac failure (dyspnoea on exertion, orthopnoea, paroxysmal nocturnal dyspnoea);
      • paroxysms of sweating and tachycardia in phaeochromocytoma.
    b The non-invasive arterial BP should be measured on a number of occasions in an attempt to rule out 'white-coat' hypertension. However, a single elevated preoperative BP has been shown to be associated with BP lability under anaesthesia.

      Do include in your examination the signs of end-organ damage (for example retinal changes can be indicative of chronicity and severity) and secondary causes (for example the abdominal bruit of renal artery stenosis or the radio-femoral delay of coarctation).

    c Hypertensive patients require the following investigations preoperatively:
      • urea, creatinine and electrolytes—to assess renal impairment;
      • ECG—to assess left ventricular hypertrophy, ischaemia and conduction defects.

29 Hypertensive patients suffer with an increase in sympathetic tone resulting in vasoconstriction and medial hypertrophy of their arterioles. Their vascular tone is poorly controlled so that anaesthesia may result in massive abrupt vasodilation. Profound vasoconstriction and hypovolaemia is often present in shocked patients as a compensatory mechanism. If this is abolished by anaesthesia, it can result in a catastrophic fall in blood pressure. In addition, in the face of hypertensive stimuli (for example intubation, pain) their BP may rise uncontrollably.

30 If surgery is continued in spite of uncontrolled hypertension, the perioperative morbidity might include MI, congestive cardiac failure (CCF), cerebrovascular accident (CVA) and renal failure.

31 Treatments to control hypertension include diuretics, beta-blockers, calcium antagonists and angiotensin-converting enzyme (ACE) inhibitors. Even though these will control hypertension they may interact with the anaesthetic, and it is important for

the anaesthetists to be aware of any concomitant medication.

32   Generally, if hypertensive patients are controlled on treatment they present the same risk as normotensive patients presenting for the same procedure.

33   Emergency operation on a patient with uncontrolled hypertension requires the following steps:

- The risks of the proposed surgical procedure must be fully but tactfully explained to the patient and his or her relatives.
- The anaesthetist should then be consulted and, ideally, the patient should be carefully monitored before and after surgery in a high-dependency unit (HDU).
- Monitoring must be continuous and the anaesthetist should be ready to give inotropes (for example dobutamine), vasoconstrictors (for example norepinephrine [noradrenaline]), or hypotensive drugs (for example labetalol, a beta-blocking agent, glyceryl trinitrate or hydralazine).

Respiratory disease

Respiratory disease is one of the most common causes of important post-operative complications and thus merits special consideration. A proper history should be taken, including whether breathlessness occurs at rest, when speaking or exercising. Always check the respiratory rate during physical examination as part of 'look, listen, feel'. Remember to consider respiratory disease in conjunction with cardiac disease for the following reasons:

- It often coexists in patients with the relevant risk factors (for example in smokers).
- Hypoxia can accentuate cardiac disease, and cardiac disease can affect respiratory status.
- The oxygen flux equation, and the importance of affecting two or more factors.

Anaesthesia and surgery have deleterious effects on respiratory function in normal patients. These effects are more likely to lead to post-operative respiratory complications in those with pre-existing lung diseases. Most anaesthetic drugs have a depressant effect on respiration. The functional residual capacity (FRC) and residual volume (RV) are reduced during anaesthesia and ventilation/perfusion matching becomes less good, resulting in a reduction in p_aO_2 and an increase in p_aCO_2. These effects cause atelectasis in dependent lung areas. Post-operatively, recovery from this is influenced by many factors, including pain, sedation, the site of surgery, residual anaesthetic drugs, abdominal distension and the supine position, all of which influence the patient's ability to cough and mobilize. Even patients with previously normal lungs suffer impairment of oxygenation for at least 48 h after abdominal surgery. This is less marked with lower abdominal surgery and worse after thoracic, thoraco-abdominal or upper abdominal procedures. In most patients after abdominal surgery these changes have resolved by the fifth or sixth post-operative day. However, they may become the focus for infection, especially if there is retention of secretions, and this can initiate the downward spiral to post-operative respiratory failure.

You will look at respiratory physiology and thoracic anatomy in STEP™ Foundation Module 3. In this section, we will consider the problems created by the patient presenting for surgery with concomitant disease.

▼

> ### Learning exercise   34
> What predisposing factors can you think of for the development of post-operative respiratory complications?

> ### Learning exercise   35
> What form would your perioperative management strategy take for a patient with significant respiratory disease?

> ### Learning exercise   36
> What would be your advice if a patient presents for surgery having had a recent upper respiratory tract infection (URTI)?

See answers to learning exercises on page 134.

It is important to liaise with the anaesthetist, chest physician and physiotherapist as appropriate. It might be that ventilation on ITU needs to be considered, in which case close discussion with the ITU is indicated. This often cannot be arranged at short notice.

Having considered some general points regarding respiratory patients let us move on to consider the main respiratory diseases we might encounter in the pre-admission clinic.

In this respiratory section we are going to cover:

- asthma;
- COPD;
- smoking;
- obesity as it relates to respiratory disease;
- steroid cover.

Asthma

Asthma is a common condition affecting some 4% of adults in the UK. It is vital that you know and understand the implications of an asthmatic patient presenting for surgery and the various modes of optimizing their treatment.

- Normally treated using bronchodilators and anti-inflammatory agents.
- Monitored using a peak flow meter—ideally >250–300 l/min preoperatively (beware of diurnal dips).
- Assess severity preoperatively including any previous ventilation.
- Operate when disease is under good control.
- Give preoperative bronchodilator therapy.
- Steroid cover required if systemic steroids have been taken for more than 2 weeks prior to surgery or for more than 1 month in the preceding year.
- Pre- and post-operative physiotherapy important.

There are a number of potential problems that might be encountered perioperatively in the controlled or uncontrolled asthmatic:

- drug interactions;
- intra-operative wheeze leading to ventilation problems and hypoxia;
- concurrent chest infections;
- post-operative hypoxia and wheeze.

The chances of any single asthmatic patient suffering from these problems can be affected significantly by your management.

Learning exercise	37

When you encounter an asthmatic patient in the preoperative clinic what symptoms should you look out for?

Learning exercise	38

In the same patient what are the significant signs?

Learning exercise	39

What investigations would you order?

Learning exercise	40

How would you manage the patient preoperatively?

See answers to learning exercises on page 134.

If an asthmatic patient presents with active disease and wheezing, the operative procedure should be delayed if at all possible. The chance of complications increases significantly.

Now try clinical case 7.

Clinical case 7

Mr Richard Maguire is a 19-year-old asthmatic in whom you have made a clinical diagnosis of acute appendicitis. He has had severe asthma since childhood which is not currently well controlled. He uses his salbutamol inhaler several times each day although he does not take his steroid inhaler regularly. He has had two courses of oral steroids this year. He has never been ventilated.

Q1 How would you assess the severity of his asthma now?

Q2 What therapy should you institute in the time available before theatre?

Q3 How will you manage him post-operatively?

Clinical case 7 answers

Q1 You would assess the severity of this patient's asthma as follows:
  - history—sleep disturbance, exercise tolerance, diurnal variation in symptoms, days off work, precipitants;
  - examination—chest deformity, wheeze;
  - investigations—peak expiratory flow rate (PEFR), pulmonary function tests (PFTs).

Q2 The following therapeutic measures should be taken before theatre:
  - continuation of his bronchodilator therapy, including the addition of nebulized salbutamol pre-theatre;
  - introduction to the physiotherapist and commencement of physiotherapy as

soon as able;

◦ steroid cover.

Q3 Post-operatively, this patient requires good pain control to allow him to co-operate fully with physiotherapy and to mobilize. He should also receive oxygen therapy, probably at least overnight, with pulse oximetry monitoring.

Answers to learning exercises

34 Predisposing factors for the development of post-operative respiratory complications include:

- site of surgery—especially upper abdominal or thoracic surgery;
- pre-existing respiratory disease—especially if current infection;
- smoking;
- obesity.

35 In a patient with significant respiratory disease, the aim of the perioperative management strategy is to minimize the complication rate by:

- adequate preoperative assessment, including investigations and blood tests;
- optimization of the patient's condition, preferably in conjunction with a chest physician;
- suitable choice of techniques (local vs. general);
- attentive post-operative supervision and management (analgesia, oxygenation, physiotherapy, etc.).

36 Surgery following a recent URTI is a very difficult area with no real hard evidence about what we should be doing. The best advice we have at the moment is that all elective surgery should be deferred for at least 1 month following bacterial or viral URTI. The evidence would suggest that the risk of desaturation, bronchospasm and post-operative infection is higher if these guidelines are ignored. If a patient is admitted as an emergency then obviously this changes things and you will have to manage as best you can. If possible defer for 1 or 2 days to allow physiotherapy and antibiotics to work if necessary.

37 The features to look for in an asthmatic patient attending the preoperative clinic are:

- duration of symptoms—is the patient recently diagnosed or has the disease been lifelong?
- exercise tolerance—is wheezing brought on by exercise and does the disease limit their exercise ability?
- recent active cold/flu/chest infection—infection within 1 month of presentation for surgery is likely to increase the chance of bronchospasm. Delay if at all possible, even if symptoms seem minimal.
- treatment—you can deduce a lot from the amount of treatment required to control symptoms, for example if steroid-dependent we can assume pretty severe disease.
- previous hospital admissions—some patients with mild disease are easily managed by GPs away from hospital. Hospital admissions ± ventilation imply disease which is less easy to control.
- smoking history—smoking and asthma is generally bad news. Patients are more

likely to suffer complications.

38 The significant signs in an asthmatic patient are:

- active wheeze—complications are more likely and patients with active symptoms should be delayed if possible. If delay is not possible then aggressive control of symptoms preop is mandatory.
- shortness of breath—implies severe disease and should be sorted out preoperatively.
- chronic asthmatics may have a hyperinflated chest.

39 Generally, in well-controlled asthmatics no specific investigations are indicated except a peak flow, which will give an instantaneous reading of airway function. The importance of investigations relates to doubt over the cause of shortness of breath, which might be irreversible (COPD) or cardiac. In this situation blood gases and lung function tests are important.

40 Preoperative management of the asthmatic patient should include the following steps.

- When admitted ensure that no deterioration in symptoms has occurred.
- Continue bronchodilator therapy around the operation. Preoperative bronchodilators help to prevent operative bronchospasm. If the patient is a severe asthmatic they might benefit from a nebulizer.
- If on steroids then prescribe intravenous steroids to cover the period of the operation.

C ☐
S ☐
R ☐

Chronic obstructive pulmonary disease

This is also a common condition but one that is more prevalent in the elderly population. It is particularly prevalent in long-term smokers, when it may be associated with significant cardiac disease. The combination may prove more problematic than each condition separately (see oxygen flux equation).

COPD is characterized mainly by airflow obstruction with cough, sputum, dyspnoea and wheeze, and the following clinical features:.

- Chronic, progressive disorder with intermittent acute exacerbations.
- Often desaturate markedly during normal sleep.
- Severity best assessed by exercise tolerance.
- Beware of right ventricular dysfunction secondary to chronic hypoxia (cor pulmonale).
- Full blood count (FBC) may reveal polycythaemia.
- Chest X-ray important as a baseline preoperatively.
- Spirometry preoperatively in all with dyspnoea on mild or moderate exercise.
- Forced expiratory volume in 1 second (FEV_1)/forced vital capacity (FVC) usually <65% and reversibility with bronchodilators minimal.
- Arterial blood gases in all with dyspnoea at rest.
- Hypoxic drive for respiration is rare.
- Treat any infective exacerbation preoperatively.
- Sputum for microbial culture and sensitivity (MCS) preoperatively will guide any post-operative antibiotic choice.
- Operate during best season.

- Physiotherapy with incentive spirometry should be started preoperatively.
- Often require prolonged oxygen and physiotherapy post-operatively.
- May benefit from postoperative epidural analgesia.

As we have seen with asthmatics, these patients may suffer problems with wheezing, which will require your attention. However, there are other problems with COPD that are perhaps less commonly associated with asthma:

- considerable sputum production leading to airway obstruction;
- irreversible airway disease;
- chronic hypoxia;
- CO_2 retention;
- associated diseases related to smoking;
- cor pulmonale;
- susceptability to acute exacerbations.

These patients require careful perioperative management to avoid respiratory failure and periods of post-operative ventilation. Weaning from post-operative ventilation can be a significant problem and therefore ventilation should be avoided at all costs.

Learning exercise	41

In COPD patients, what symptoms and signs lead you to establish the severity of their disease?

Learning exercise	42

a   What investigations help you in this?

b   Look at Fig. 1.4.3. What abnormalities does it show?

Fig. 1.4.3

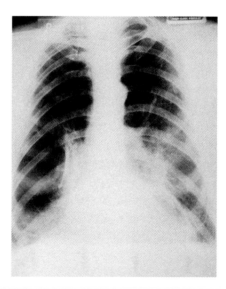

Learning exercise	43

What can be done perioperatively to reduce the risk to the patient?

| Learning exercise | 44 |

How may blood gases help in the preparation of the patient?

| Learning exercise | 45 |

How may oxygen be given to a patient with COPD?

Smoking

Smoking can affect the perioperative course in two ways:

1 directly as a result of a reduction in Hb oxygen-carrying capacity;

2 indirectly by causing diseases of the cardiovascular, respiratory and immune systems.

Smoking has multiple deleterious effects in the perioperative period:

- Increases the risk of post-operative respiratory complications sixfold.
- Carboxyhaemoglobin may reduce the oxygen-carrying capacity of blood by 25%.

It should be remembered that carbon monoxide (CO) and nicotine are cleared from the body in 12–24 h. Stopping smoking for this short period of time can significantly reduce the chances of complications. Six to eight weeks of cessation required to unequivocally improve bronchoconstriction and reduce mucus secretion.

| Learning exercise | 46 |

List the effects of smoking on the respiratory and cardiac systems.

| Learning exercise | 47 |

How does smoking affect the amount of oxygen carried in the blood?

Try to stop patients smoking before surgery—every little bit helps to smooth the perioperative course.

Answers to learning exercises

41   In COPD the following symptoms and signs indicate the severity of disease.

Symptoms

- Cough productive of green sputum suggesting acute exacerbation.
- Shortness of breath (SOB) on minimal exercise or rest suggesting minimal respiratory reserve.
- Steroid dependence.
- Continuing to smoke.

Signs

- Lung crepitations.
- Clubbing.
- Cyanosis.
- Jugular venous pulse raised/hepatomegaly suggesting cor pulmonale.

42   a   Investigations that can help in assessing the severity of COPD include:

- ECG—signs of right ventricular strain/axis deviation.
- Chest X-ray—may show hyperexpansion or prominent pulmonary arteries, but not good at predicting severity of disease.
- blood gases on air—show the degree of hypoxia and CO_2 retention. However you should never take oxygen off a patient who requires urgent blood gas analysis!
- lung function tests—reduced FEV_1/FVC ratio.

b   Figure 1.4.3 is a chest X-ray of a patient who is suffering from severe COPD. It shows the following abnormalities:

- decreased parenchymal lung shadows, with increased radiolucency in the peripheral lung fields;
- a flattening of the diaphragm;
- increased lung capacity.

43   Various measures can be taken, both preoperatively and post-operatively, to reduce the risks to the patient with COPD.

Preoperative

- Operate during a time of year when acute exacerbations are less likely, for example summer months.
- Stop patient smoking preoperatively for at least a few weeks.
- Careful assessment of appropriateness of planned procedure in view of increased risks to patient because of COPD. This must include proper counselling of patient.
- Decide upon which form of anaesthetic is most appropriate, for example general anaesthetic, regional or local anaesthetic to minimize respiratory depression.

Avoid ventilation, if general anaesthetic is necessary—they may be difficult to wean.

- Preoperative physiotherapy, especially if sputum production is a problem, to teach patient the importance of deep expiration and expectoration.
- Use nebulizers preoperatively.
- Perform blood gases, lung function tests and sputum cultures, where appropriate.
- If there is preoperative infection, antibiotics must be given, based, if possible, on a sputum culture.

Post-operative

- Adequate pain relief avoiding opiates and NSAIDs (if aspirin sensitive).

Of particular value are patient-controlled analgesia (PCA), epidural analgesia and efficient local blockade, for example ilio-inguinal block and cryodestruction of intercostal nerves during thoracotomy.

- Post-operative physiotherapy will be given to prevent atelectasis and infection.
- Close vigilance for infection and treat early if deteriorating.
- Proper delivery of oxygen, i.e. 28% oxygen via a Venti mask at 4 l/min. In addition, humidification and nebulized bronchodilators may be necessary.

Remember to take care when administering oxygen to a patient with COPD:

- Avoid too high a concentration of inspired oxygen.
- Some patients with COPD rely on a hypoxic drive for respiration, as they are

constantly subjected to an increased alveolar carbon dioxide level. Thus, removing the hypoxic drive by giving high concentrations of inspired oxygen may have disastrous effects on the patient, with subsequent respiratory failure.

- One method of diluting the oxygen flow to safer levels is to employ the Venturi principle. Here, the oxygen flow is streamlined through a plastic tube into a mask, which has holes in it. The flow of oxygen 'draws' atmospheric air into the face mask through the holes, so diluting the oxygen concentration in the mask before it reaches the patient's lungs.

- Since it is hypoxia that is largely responsible for myocardial ischaemia and CVA, it is acceptable to accept marginally high p_aCO_2 levels if these are associated with a 'safe' p_aO_2.

- Humidified oxygen delivery prevents the patient's airways from becoming dried out with consequent difficulty in expectoration. Nasal oxygen delivered through two small plastic ports placed at the nares achieves the same effect. It is vital to realize that low p_aO_2 happens in elderly patients and delivery of post-operative transnasal oxygen for several days is important.

- With respiratory failure, ventilation and tracheostomy may be necessary on occasions.

44   Blood gases taken on air help us to establish the severity of disease and the amount of CO_2 retention:

- a pO_2 on air of <7 kPa suggests significant disease and any compromise in respiratory function could be catastrophic—particularly bad if CO_2 is raised.

- CO_2 >7 kPa implies retention of CO_2 and consideration for ventilation post-op.

- Also look at the bicarbonate. Patients with a respiratory acidosis will have a compensatory metabolic alkalosis and high bicarbonate. This suggests long-standing disease and a high likelihood of requiring ventilation.

45   If the patient with COPD is not retaining CO_2, giving oxygen should not be a problem. It should be stated that CO_2 retention is uncommon so be prepared to give oxygen freely. If CO_2 is being retained then the central nervous system (CNS) chemoreceptors adjust and the patient loses the ability for CO_2 to control ventilation. They therefore rely on a hypoxic drive, which might be abolished by the administration of high concentrations of oxygen. Oxygen should therefore be given through a fixed-concentration controlled Venturi mask at 24% or 28% depending on the response of the gases. Remember that in these patients we are not looking for supranormal pO_2 levels. They are used to a pO_2 of 6 or 7 kPa, so don't try to get it to 10 or 15 kPa.

46   The principal effects of smoking on the respiratory and cardiovascular systems are:

- Respiratory system
  - reduced ciliary motility;
  - sputum production;
  - small airway narrowing;
  - increased airway reactivity.
- Cardiovascular system
  - IHD;

C ☐
S ☐
R ☐

- hypertension;
- cerebrovascular disease.

47 Smoking produces CO for which Hb has a greater affinity than oxygen. This CO therefore binds to the oxygen-binding sites preventing oxygen from binding. In addition, the ability of Hb to give up its oxygen to the tissues is reduced (i.e. tissue oxygen delivery is reduced) as the Hb dissociation curve is displaced to the left.

Obesity and respiratory function

Obesity can also have a profound effect on respiratory function, particularly in the post-operative period. There is an epidemic of obesity in the Western World. Within the UK, by 1998 obesity (defined as a BMI >30) was affecting 19% of the population (21% of women, 17% of men), a proportion which has have trebled over the last 20 years.

Morbid obesity is defined as a patient with a BMI >40 kg/m². If morbidity is already present, then the risks are equivalent to patients with BMI >35 kg/m². The complications arise from two sources:

1 the direct effect of the obesity on the respiratory system;
2 the co-morbidity associated with the obesity.

The effects on the respiratory system include:

- a reduction in vital capacity (VC) and FRC;
- increased work of breathing;
- basal atelectasis leading to hypoxia;
- airway narrowing;
- respiratory disadvantage worsened by supine position.

The co-morbidity includes:

- cardiovascular disease resulting from an increased strain on the heart;
- diabetes;
- gastric incompetence resulting in increased risk of aspiration;
- greater risk of DVT;
- difficulty in venous access;
- airway mangement problems in the perioperative period, for example sleep apnoea syndrome.

Learning exercise	48

What problems might you encounter in theatre and recovery with a morbidly obese patient?

Learning exercise	49

What problems might you encounter once the patient has returned to the ward?

Learning exercise	50

How are obese patients best managed on the wards?

See answers to learning exercises on page 143.

Steroids and respiratory disease

Bear in mind that there are two main reasons why someone may be taking steroids in conjunction with respiratory disease:

1 to cover an acute exacerbation;

2 as part of their regular preventative medication. This will be either as inhaled steroids (for example beclomethasone) or oral for severe COPD. Inhaled steroids of less than 1600 µg/day have minimal systemic effect.

Steroids are commonly used in the treatment of respiratory diseases, but remember:

- systemic steroids cause adrenal suppression (>10 mg/day of prednisolone or equivalent);
- inhaled steroids are not taken up significantly systemically;
- failure to use steroid cover perioperatively when indicated can, very rarely, result in an Addisonian crisis and death;
- steroid cover advised for patients on systemic steroids for more than 2 weeks prior to surgery or if discontinued within 3 months of surgery.

The quantity of steroid is tailored to the degree of stress imposed by the operation. Table 13 gives a suggested regime for oral steroid cover perioperatively:

Table 13: Perioperative regime for oral steroid cover

Procedure	Suggested steroid cover
Minor diagnostic procedures	Single-dose hydrocortisone 25 mg i.v./i.m. preop
Intermediate operations	Hydrocortisone 25 mg i.v./i.m. preop, then 25 mg 6 hourly for 24 h
Major operations	Hydrocortisone 25 mg i.v. 6 hourly for 72 h starting preop

N.B: Continue for longer if there is further 'stress' or infection.

Many published regimes continue to advocate much higher replacement doses than above. There is no evidence to support this approach and excess steroid administration may in fact be harmful. Steroid replacement therapy is generally not problematic. Clinical case 7 covered this topic.

Investigations relevant to respiratory disease

With regard to investigations, there are a number that provide valuable information about the respiratory state whatever the pathology. These are explored in the next set of learning exercises.

Learning exercise	51

What blood tests are indicated in patients with respiratory disease presenting for surgery?

Learning exercise	52

How may a chest X-ray help in the assessment of the severity of a patient's respiratory state?

When would you order pulmonary function tests and what information might you gain from them?

See answers to learning exercises on page 143.

Now try clinical case 8:

Clinical case 8

Mrs Selina Johnstone is a 71-year-old smoker who suffers from COPD. She presents at your preoperative assessment clinic in January because she is booked for a total knee replacement for the treatment of her osteoarthritis. She tells you that although she can normally manage to walk 100 m slowly before becoming breathless, over the last week or so she has been confined to the house and has been coughing up increased quantities of sputum. She has not been sleeping well. She is overweight with a BMI of 30.

Q1   What are your concerns about this case?

Q2   What do you propose to do about them?

The case is delayed until such time as the symptoms are better, and she has completed a course of antibiotics and physiotherapy to clear her chest. She returns in the summer, still smoking and overweight. Her exercise tolerance is back to her best.

Q3   What do you do this time?

Q4   What anaesthetic techniques might best suit her?

Clinical case 8 answers

Q1   The concerns are:
  ¬ age 71 suffering from COPD;
  ¬ poor exercise tolerance at best;
  ¬ still smoking;
  ¬ active chest infection.
  ¬ worsening exercise tolerance;
  ¬ overweight.

Q2   In the light of these concerns you should:
  ¬ delay her elective surgery—she is at high risk;
  ¬ advise a course of antibiotics;
  ¬ advise her to stop smoking;
  ¬ advise her to lose weight.

Q3   She is probably as good as she can be now. There is little to be gained from further postponement. Admit her, perform routine blood tests, blood gases and ECG, and consider PFTs to fully assess the state of her COPD.

Q4   She would probably benefit from a regional anaesthetic technique to avoid the use of respiratory depressant general anaesthetic. Ideally this would be an epidural so that analgesia could be carried into the post-op period thereby avoiding opiates.

Answers to learning exercises

Obesity and respiratory function

48   The morbidly obese patient can pose problems with:

- venous access;
- intubation and airway control;
- gastric reflux;
- positioning;
- moving patient;
- nerve pressure injuries;
- ventilation;
- surgical access;
- non-invasive BP measurement;
- oxygenation after extubation;
- positioning in recovery;
- analgesia.

49   Various problems might be encountered when a morbidly obese patient is returned to the ward:

- hypoxia from basal atelectasis;
- sputum retention from inadequate cough
- hypoventilation (multifactorial);
- DVT;
- analgesia problems;
- wound infection.

50   The following steps can help in managing the obese patient on the ward:

- consider HDU admission after major procedures;
- sit patient up;
- administer local anaesthetic if applicable;
- give oxygen for 48 h;
- continue heparin;
- early mobilization.

Steroids and respiratory disease

51   The following blood tests are indicated in patients with respiratory disease presenting for surgery:

- FBC
  - anaemia will worsen respiratory symptoms;
  - polycythaemia as a response to chronic hypoxia increases the risk of thromboembolism;
  - a raised white cell count may indicate an infective exacerbation.
- Urea and electrolytes (U & Es)
  - patients often take a diuretic, which would have an effect on the electrolytes.
- Arterial blood gases (ABGs)
  - perform on all patients with dyspnoea at rest;
  - useful baseline for chronic respiratory conditions;

- can identify those patients dependent on hypoxic drive for respiration;
- significant risk of post-operative respiratory failure if:
  - p_aCO_2 >6.7 kPa (50 mmHg),
  - p_aO_2 <8 kPa (60 mmHg).

52 Chest radiography is not especially useful in assessing the severity of respiratory disease. It is a poor indicator of functional impairment, and is usually performed as a baseline in to permit comparison with post-operative films.

53 The indications and useful findings of pulmonary function tests are as follows:

- Recommended for all patients with severe dyspnoea on mild to moderate exertion; may help to distinguish between 'cardiac' breathlessness and 'respiratory' breathlessness.
- Peak expiratory flow rate (PEFR) used for monitoring asthmatics.
- Used to assess response to bronchodilators.
- FEV_1/FVC ratio usually <65% in obstructive lung diseases.

C ☐
S ☐
R ☐

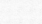

Diabetes mellitus

Diabetes mellitus is a disorder of sugar metabolism. The overall prevalence of diabetes is 2%; however in the 'surgical' population of 60–80 year olds, the true prevalence is >10%. Diabetic patients present the surgeon with two main management problems:

1. the perioperative control of blood sugar and the metabolic consequences of poor control;
2. problems related to the complications of the disease.

Learning exercise	54

Why is it important to maintain good control of blood sugar perioperatively?

Learning exercise	55

List the complications of diabetes.

Learning exercise	56

From your list of complications, what are the particular risks of anaesthesia and surgery in a diabetic patient?

Learning exercise	57

What drugs can interfere with the control of blood sugar?

Learning exercise	58

What are the treatment options for diabetes?

Learning exercise	59

How would you screen a diabetic patient for autonomic neuropathy at the bedside?

▼

Learning exercise   60

With reference to theatre list order, why are diabetic patients usually placed first on the operating list?

See answers to learning exercises on page 148.

Management of a diabetic patient presenting for surgery

From the history, examination and investigations, the severity and type of diabetes and its control need to be assessed. All except life-saving emergency surgery in the poorly controlled diabetic should be delayed until hyperglycaemia, dehydration and acidosis are corrected (NB: diabetic acidosis may mimic an acute abdomen). Furthermore, the patient should be assessed for complications related to the diabetes.

The treatment regime chosen to manage a diabetic patient presenting for surgery is dictated by:

- the nature of the surgery;
- whether the patient has Type 1 or Type 2 diabetes;
- the quality of control of the diabetes.

Minor surgery can be defined as surgery in which the patient is expected to eat and drink within 4 h of the operation. All other surgery is defined as major surgery. If the random blood sugar on admission is greater than 10 mmol/l then treat as major surgery.

Learning exercise   61

What preoperative investigations would you order for a diabetic patient?

Learning exercise   62

Outline your management of two patients who have both been admitted for cholecystectomy:
a A patient with diabetes controlled by diet alone or hypoglycaemic drugs.
b A patient with diabetes controlled by insulin.

Learning exercise   63

What is a sliding scale insulin infusion? Write down an example of an insulin and dextrose infusion regimen for a fit adult.

See answers to learning exercises on page 148.

Now try clinical cases 9 and 10:

Clinical case 9

At the preoperative assessment clinic you see Rashida Khan, a 47-year-old woman who has Type 2 diabetes. She is booked to have a breast lump excision under general anaesthesia. You learn that she is relatively fit and well although she does suffer from hypertension. Her regular medications are glipizide and enalapril. She has had diabetes for 2 years and is well controlled on tablets. A random blood glucose stick test measurement is 8 mmol/l.

Q1 What instructions are you going to give to this woman about taking her regular

▼

medication prior to admission?

Q2   How are you planning to control her diabetes during her admission?

This woman is admitted on the morning of the operation. A blood glucose stick test reveals a level of 14 mmol/l.

Q3   How does this alter your management plan?

Clinical case 9 answers

Q1   A breast lump excision is a relatively minor procedure which should require a short duration of general anaesthesia. You would expect that the patient would be able to eat and drink within 4 h. As her diabetes seems to be well controlled it would seem reasonable to continue with her normal medication until the day of operation.

Q2   On the day of operation omit oral hypoglycaemic agents and check her blood glucose stick test, and continue to do so. Continue to measure blood glucose stick test every 2 h post-operatively until she is eating and drinking. She should be listed first on the operating list and should be given instructions regarding starvation times.

Q3   If, on the morning of her operation, blood glucose stick test gives a measurement of 14 mmol/l then:
- repeat the blood glucose stick test;
- if the reading is still >10 mmol/l then set up an insulin infusion;
- measure the blood glucose stick test 2-hourly and post-operatively when she is eating and drinking, stop the insulin infusion and restart oral therapy;
- measure blood glucose stick tests 4–8-hourly.

Clinical case 10

Robert Miller is 30 years old and has diabetes. He presents with a 2-day history of vomiting and right iliac fossa pain. An acute appendicitis is suspected. You are asked to admit him and prepare him for theatre.

Q1   What information do you need to manage his diabetes appropriately?

You learn that he has had Type 1 diabetes for 10 years and is normally well controlled on regular subcutaneous insulin injections. He attends a diabetic clinic and is unaware of any diabetic-related complications. He has been unwell for 2 days and has only tolerated a few sips of water today. He tells you his blood glucose stick test readings are high.

Q2   What in particular do you look for on examination?

On examination you notice the smell of ketones. He looks dehydrated:
- Heart rate: 115 b.p.m.
- BP: 90/40 mmHg
- Temperature: 38.6 °C
- Respiratory rate: 20 breaths/min

He has not passed any urine since admission.

Q3   What investigations are you going to order?

You receive the following results:

Table 14: Robert Miller's test results

Haematology	Biochemistry	Blood gases
Hb, 14.5	Urea, 14.4	pH, 7.21
WCC, 19.1	Cr, 84	pco_2, 2.9
Platelets, 190	Na, 134	po_2, 12.6 (on air)
	K, 3.7	HCO_3, 15
	Glucose, 16	Base excess, −15

Q4   Comment on these results.

Q5   How are you going to manage this patient?

Clinical case 10 answers

Q1   In order to manage his diabetes appropriately you would want to know:
- The type of diabetes.
- What treatment he is on.
- How well his diabetes is controlled.
- History of complications.
- History of his current illness.
- How long he has been unwell.
- His fluid intake/balance.

Q2   The particular signs to look for on examination are:
- Smell of ketones, level of consciousness.
- Degree of hydration—tongue, skin turgor, etc.
- Vital signs—heart rate, BP, temperature, urine output.

Q3   You would order the following investigations:
- FBC
- U & E
- ABG
- Blood sugar estimation
- Urinalysis for ketones
- blood glucose stick test
- Blood cultures
- Urine for culture

Q4   The results show that this gentleman has become septic. He is dehydrated and has developed a metabolic acidosis. His blood sugar is poorly controlled.

Q5   Management of this patient would entail the following measures:
- Inform senior surgical colleagues about the patient and make arrangements for theatre.
- Inform the anaesthetist.
- Set up intravenous access.
- Start rapid infusion of normal saline.
- Urinary catheter.

- Give further intravenous fluid challenges according to vital signs and urine output.
- Set up a dextrose/insulin infusion and prescribe a sliding scale.
- Correct serum potassium.
- Consider a central line but the anaesthetist may prefer this to be done in theatre.

Answers to learning exercises

Diabetes mellitus

54   It is important to control the diabetic's blood sugar perioperatively to prevent hypoglycaemia or hyperglycaemia. A target blood sugar of 5–7 mmol/l is appropriate.

There is a risk of intra-operative hypoglycaemia in those patients taking long-acting oral hypoglycaemic agents or insulin. Under general anaesthesia the signs of hypoglycaemia would be masked and this could have potentially disastrous consequences for brain function. The endocrine response to hypoglycaemia, for example release of glucagon and epinephrine (adrenaline), is reduced during anaesthesia.

Equally, hyperglycaemia should be avoided perioperatively as this may lead to the development of diabetic ketoacidosis (NB: inhalational anaesthetic agents increase blood sugar). Good control has also been shown to reduce wound infection and outcome in the critically ill.

55   The complications of diabetes are significant with a reduction in life expectancy of 5–10 years. They can broadly be divided as follows:

- macrovascular disease;
  - IHD and (cardiomyopathy);
  - peripheral vascular disease (PVD) (15%–60%) (foot ulcers);
  - cerebrovascular disease;
- microvascular;
  - nephropathy (albuminurea, hypertension, renal failure);
  - neuropathy (many including autonomic and symmetrical distal polyneuropathy);
  - diabetic eye disease (cataract and retinopathy);
- others;
  - susceptibility to any infection;
  - hypertension (more 'associated' in renal disease and metabolic syndrome);
  - respiratory (fall in FEV_1 and FRC).

56   Certain complications of diabetes pose particular risks during anaesthesia and surgery:

- Vascular disease will increase the risk of cardiac and cerebral complications with an increased risk of MI and CVA. Hypotension is poorly tolerated, particularly post-operatively.
- Autonomic neuropathy may result in sudden tachycardia, hypotension and unexpected cardiac arrest (NB: hypertension is the strongest correlate of autonomic neuropathy). It also causes delayed gastric emptying and increases the risk of aspiration (this is one reason why the anaesthetist may prefer to opt for a regional or local technique).

▼

- Cardiomyopathy will lead to ventricular dysfunction.
- Nephropathy—there is increased risk of acute renal failure and UTI.
- Infection—sepsis and poor wound healing are a major cause of perioperative morbidity.
- Respiratory—the incidence of chest infection and chronic obstructive airways disease is increased, particularly in obese patients.
- Retinopathy—there is a risk of vitreous haemorrhage during hypertensive manoeuvres, for example intubation.

57 Corticosteroids and thiazide diuretics can interfere with the control of blood sugar.

58 The treatment options for diabetes are:

- diet;
- oral hypoglycaemics:
  - sulphonylureas (glipizide, gliclazide)—stimulate the production of glucose by the liver;
  - biguanides (metformin)—increase tissue utilization and reduce glucose production and intestinal glucose absorption. Complication is lactic acidosis (very rare).
- glitazones (rosiglitazone, pioglitazone)—sensitize tissues to insulin-reducing insulin resistance;
- meglitanides (nateglinide, repaglinide)—similar to sulphonylureas but more rapid onset with shorter duration;
- insulin.

59 Bedside indications of autonomic neuropathy in the diabetic patient include:

- postural drop in BP greater than 30 mmHg;
- reduced heart rate response to the Valsalva manoeuvre;
- loss of beat to beat variation in heart rate.

60 Diabetic patients are preferably listed first on the operating list to minimize the duration of starvation and hence the metabolic disturbance. The ideal is for the patient to present for surgery with normal blood sugar and normal glycogen stores.

61 The following preoperative investigations are relevant for the diabetic patient:

- random blood sugar estimation;
- 12-lead ECG.
- urea and electrolyte estimation;
- urinalysis 4-hourly for ketones and sugar throughout admission;
- Blood glucose stick testing 4-hourly preoperatively if insulin-dependent Type 1;
- Blood glucose stick testing 8-hourly preoperatively if non-insulin-dependent Type 2.

There are a variety of insulin/dextrose regimes used in different hospitals but they are all aiming to supply glucose and insulin in a suitable volume of intravenous fluid to maintain normal blood glucose and limit the production of ketones. If you recall that dextrose/insulin is a treatment for hyperkalaemia then it follows that it will be necessary to monitor serum potassium levels and supplement as needed (some regimes include potassium in the infusions). Separate dextrose/insulin infusions offer more flexibility and are 'usual' in most centres.

62 Management relevant to all diabetic patients:

- Explain the management of diabetes over the operative period to the patient.
- Do an ECG in middle-aged diabetic patients preoperatively because of the risk of heart disease.
- Achieve the best possible control before surgery (NB: glucose levels will be higher with sepsis, stress and inactivity).
- Arrange for the patient's operation to be at the start of the list.

  a The management of patients on dietary control of diabetes or oral hypoglycaemic drugs (i.e. 85% of diabetic patients) entails the following measures:

  ⊓ Patients should stop their tablets on the day of surgery (stop chlorpropamide or similar compounds 48 h before operation because they are long acting).

  ⊓ Diabetes, especially if well controlled, is not a contraindication to day surgery procedures.

  ⊓ Place the patient first on the list and set up an intravenous infusion of dextrose saline 1 litre 10 hourly.

  ⊓ Monitor glucose levels regularly, with blood glucose stick testing 1–3-hourly (once-hourly if the patient is unconscious).

  ⊓ Deliver insulin, by sliding scale, to control blood glucose within normal range, if necessary.

  ⊓ Resume oral hypoglycaemics when allowed to eat and check blood glucose stick testing 6-hourly before meals.

  b Management of the insulin-controlled diabetic coming to surgery involves the following:

  ⊓ Omit long-acting insulin the night before the operation and the early-morning insulin on the operation day; put up 5% dextrose to run 8-hourly.

  ⊓ Intravenous lactate solutions do not need to be avoided and may actually be the solutions of choice.

  ⊓ Blood glucose stick testing should be checked preoperatively, hourly during the operation, and 4-hourly after operation. Also check potassium if it is a long operation.

  ⊓ Keep the blood glucose levels within safe limits (5–7 mmol/l is ideal) over the perioperative period.

  ⊓ Design a sliding scale using Human Velosulin® or Actrapid® 2-hourly.

  ⊓ Although sliding scales are convenient, there must be a constant review of the diabetic control. It is safer to keep the blood glucose level slightly higher than normal, especially if control is brittle.

  ⊓ Use a flexible method of administration when giving the glucose and insulin.

▼

Ideally, the two should be run in separately, so that the doses may be independently adjusted. The insulin and glucose may also be mixed in the same infusion bag (i.e. 10% glucose, 500 ml containing 50 units of soluble insulin, and 40–50 mmol of KCl), infused at the rate of 100 ml/h.

⅂ When oral feeding recommences, return to the original insulin dosage, and check the blood glucose stick testing 6-hourly before meals.

⅂ Take particular care to avoid sepsis. Watch for it and treat promptly.

63   A sliding scale insulin infusion is a prescription for intravenous insulin that varies in its rate of administration depending on the blood glucose stick testing.

Insulin/dextrose infusion regime for a fit adult is as follows:

- Give 2 litres 5% dextrose over 24 h.
- Prepare 50 units of Actrapid® insulin made up to 50 ml with normal saline.
- Infuse using a syringe pump.
- Attach to a non-return valve/dedicated intravenous line.
- Insulin sliding scale.

Table 15: Insulin sliding scale regimen

Blood glucose (mmol/l)	Insulin (units/h)
<3	0 (call doctor)
3.1–4.0	0.5
4.1–6.0	1
6.1–9.0	2
9.1–11.0	3
11.1–13.0	4
13.1–15.0	5
15.1–20.0	6
>20	8 (call doctor)

Deep vein thrombosis

As mentioned in preceding sections, you should be conversant with local policies on thromboembolic prophylaxis. In the section we shall learn about the principles which guide the formulation of those local policies.

Aetiology and risk factors

The approximate incidence of DVT is 50 per 100 000 of the population, with the incidence of pulmonary embolization (PE) being approximately half of this rate. Some 20%–50% of patients undergoing a major general surgical or orthopaedic procedure will develop a DVT.

Patients at increased risk for DVT and PE are:

- those with a previous history of venous thrombosis;
- surgical patients following major abdominal, pelvic and orthopaedic procedures;
- older patients;
- sufferers from varicose veins;
- obese patients;
- surgical patients who have had a long duration of surgery;

C ☐
S ☐
R ☐

- patients with blood disorders such as polycythaemia, thrombocythaemia and coagulation disorders;
- patients who have had bed rest of over 4 days;
- pregnant patients;
- recipients of high-dose oestrogen therapy;
- malignancy;
- patients with heart failure;
- patients who have had a recent MI;
- patients with infection;
- patients with inflammatory bowel disease.

Thromboprophylaxis

The incidence of DVT can be significantly reduced by the appropriate use of prophylaxis in patients at risk. There are several different methods of prophylaxis and protocol varies from hospital to hospital. In 1992, a Working Party of the Royal Colleges of Anaesthetists and Surgeons of England published the THRIFT guidelines for DVT prophylaxis. These stated that all patients should be assessed for clinical risk, including those for regional and local anaesthesia, and should receive prophylaxis according to their degree of risk.

Protocol for general surgery

All general surgery in-patients should be assessed for clinical risk, including those for regional or local anaesthesia. All patients receive prophylaxis according to their degree of risk until discharge at least.

Thromboprophylaxis can be administered using physical methods and pharmacological agents. It is important to remember the possibility of thrombophilia both in risk factor assessment and in the diagnosis of DVT. Remember to screen for this by taking both a a personal and family history. Table 16 is an example of one local policy for thromboprophylaxis.

Table 16: Thromboembolic risk prophylaxis

Risk	prophylaxis
Low	
Minor surgery (<30 min); no risk factors other than age	Early mobilization only
Major surgery (>30 min), age <40 years	
Moderate	
Major surgery, age >40 years	Subcutaneous low molecular weight heparin (LMWH); dosage according to preparation
Minor surgery with previous DVT/PE	
High	
Major pelvic/abdominal surgery for cancer	Subcutaneous LMWH; dosage according to preparation
Major surgery with previous DVT/PE	Subcutaneous heparin 5000 U 8-hourly plus graduated compression stockings
Major lower limb amputation	
Acute lower limb paralysis	
Acute abdominal surgery >40 years	

Now work through the following learning exercises:

Learning exercise	64

Venous thromboembolism is an important and indeed potentially preventable phenomenon. Identify local and general risk factors at each of the following stages and indicate the action you would take to reduce risk in the preoperative and operative periods.

Learning exercise	65

List some physical methods of thromboprophylaxis.

Learning exercise	66

List the pharmacological agents used in DVT prophylaxis and describe their actions.

Answers to learning exercises

64   The risk factors for venous thromboembolism at the different stages, and the possible preventive measures, are given in Table 17.

Table 17: Risk factors for venous thromboembolism

Stage	Local risk factors	Preventive action	General risk factors	Preventive action
(a) Preoperative		None	Smoking	Advice cessation
	Congenital venous abnormality	None	Obesity	Advise weight loss
			Pregnancy	Consider delaying non-urgent surgery until after delivery
			Oral contraceptive pill	Stop 6 weeks before surgery
			Previous DVT or PE	In all cases
			Neoplasia	TED stockings
			Female sex + age >40 years	(except if significant peripheral vascular disease) Administer low-dose or low molecular weight heparin, starting at time of premedication and/or I.V. dextran 70
			Preoperative immobility	
			Trauma cases	
			Pre-existing cardiovascular disease	
(b) Operative	Venous surgery	Minimize trauma to veins	Operation >30 min	Expeditious surgery Inflatable leggings
	Sepsis			Electrical calf stimulation

Stage	Local risk factors	Preventive action	General risk factors	Preventive action
	Major pelvic and hip surgery			?I.V. dextran
	Knee replacement surgery			

65 Physical methods of thromboprophylaxis include:

- low-voltage stimulation of calf muscles intraoperatively;
- pneumatic calf compression intra-operatively;
- elastic graduated compression stockings;
- early ambulation.

66 The pharmacological agents used for DVT prophylaxis are listed below.

- Heparin/LMWH. Standard or unfractionated heparin and LMWH have been shown conclusively to prevent venous thromboembolism. They facilitate the action of antithrombin III to inhibit the active forms of clotting factors IX, X, XI and XII. Studies have also shown that a single daily dose of LMWH is at least as effective as heparin given 8- or 12-hourly because of its longer duration of action. Significant perioperative bleeding is markedly reduced with LMWH.

- Dextran intravenously. This is used perioperatively to expand plasma volume, which decreases venous stasis. It also alters normal platelet adhesiveness.

Oral anticoagulants, for example warfarin. These antagonize the action of vitamin K in the liver and inhibit the synthesis of factors II, VII, IX and X. However, prophylactic use of oral anticoagulation is associated with a high risk of major haemorrhage perioperatively.

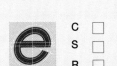

C ☐
S ☐
R ☐

Surgical management of the pregnant patient

Pregnancy induces many physiological and anatomical changes in the mother. These may alter or suppress a disease process and make clinical assessment of the patient difficult.

Always consider:

- the effect of the disease on the pregnancy;
- the effect of the pregnancy on the disease.

When investigating and treating a pregnant patient bear in mind the well-being of the fetus and the mother.

Improved antenatal follow-up and a better understanding of pregnancy has drastically decreased the maternal mortality rate. However, when a pregnant patient presents with a coexisting surgical problem she is at much higher risk than if she were not pregnant. The consequences of missing pathology or operating unnecessarily can be catastrophic for both the mother and the fetus.

Assessment

Both the history and the physical examination can be difficult to interpret in the pregnant patient. Non-specific complaints, which are common during pregnancy, are also a common presenting feature of surgical pathology. The normal physiological changes of pregnancy (see learning exercises) can make special investigations unreliable. The condition of the fetus and mother will have to be assessed and reassessed, before making any management decisions. Some of the severe medical conditions of pregnancy may present in a very similar way to surgical pathology and must, if possible, be ruled out before considering a surgical diagnosis.

There is concern about exposing an immature fetus to excessive radiation, and interpreting X-rays of the abdomen, especially in advanced pregnancy, is difficult. Other forms of imaging may be more useful. Ultrasound scanning may be very useful as it has minimal effects on the fetus and may help differentiate surgical from non-surgical pathology.

Repeated examination by a skilled clinician with an understanding of the limitations of the examination and of the disease processes in pregnancy, remains the most useful method of assessing pregnant patients.

Clinical management

Missed surgical pathology can cause premature labour, with a high fetal and maternal morbidity. A combined team of obstetricians and surgeons should manage these patients. The condition of all patients should be optimized prior to surgery with careful attention to fluid status and pulmonary function. They are at high risk of pulmonary complications, including aspiration, pulmonary embolism and post-operative hypoxia. Maintaining normal maternal physiology will minimize the adverse effects on the fetus. Once a surgical diagnosis is made, rapid intervention by a skilled surgical team is required.

Learning exercise	67

Describe the physiological changes of pregnancy with special reference to the following systems:

a Cardiovascular.

b Respiratory.

c Haematological.

d Renal.

e GI tract.

Learning exercise	68

Outline the special considerations when prescribing drugs to a pregnant patient.

Learning exercise	69

What are the important aspects of managing the pregnant patient with surgical disease?

See answers to learning exercises on page 157.

Now try clinical case 11:

Clinical case 11

Mrs Reid is 31 years old. She is day 2 post-elective Caesarean section. She was previously well and had a normal pregnancy. You are asked to give a surgical opinion as she has developed abdominal distension and is vomiting.

Q1 What are the significant positive or negative features in her history?

On examination she is 37.8 °C. Her abdomen is distended and tender over the lower abdomen. She has no bowel sounds. The chart records that she has vomited four times in the last 2 h. The rest of the examination is normal.

Q2 What is your differential diagnosis at present?

Q3 What investigations would you request?

Q4 How would you manage her while her investigations were completed and a diagnosis established?

Clinical case 11 answers

Q1 The significant features of her history are:
  ¬ previous normal pregnancy;
  ¬ Day 2 post-elective Caesarean section;
  ¬ acute distension and vomiting—features of paralytic ileus or obstruction.

Q2 A temperature of 37.8 °C is abnormal in the post-partum patient. Common causes would be breast engorgement, UTI or DVT of the calves.

Possible causes of her abdominal signs and symptoms are post-operative ileus, severe constipation or intra-abdominal collection.

Q3 You would request the following investigations:
  ¬ FBC.
  ¬ U & Es.
  ¬ Urine microscopy.
  ¬ Plain abdominal X-ray.
  ¬ Abdominal ultrasound.
  ¬ Ultrasound of the calves if clinically suspect.

Q4 While waiting for completion of the investigations and diagnosis, you would institute the following measures:
  ¬ Nasogastric tube.
  ¬ IVI fluids.
  ¬ DVT prophylaxis.
  ¬ Analgesia.

Answers to learning exercises

Surgical management of the pregnant patient

67 The physiological changes occurring during pregnancy are numerous but some of the more common ones are listed below.

a Cardiovascular:
- raised CO, stroke volume (SV), and HR;
- Oedema (from raised venous pressure);
- reduced systemic vascular resistance (SVR);
- systolic murmur (ejection systolic murmur at the left sternal edge).
- Respiratory:
- SOB (pulmonary capillary engorgement);
- respiratory alkalosis (increased minute ventilation);
- rapid desaturation (due to decreased FRC and increased oxygen consumption).

b Haematological:
- physiological anaemia (increased blood and plasma volume, relative haemodilution) result in increased iron and folate requirement;
- up to 1500 ml blood loss is usually tolerated by a healthy parturient;
- hypercoagulable state: increased clotting factors;
- decreased serum albumin;
- increased WCC with a neutrophilia.

c Renal:
- increased glomerular filtration rate (GFR);
- plasma urea decreased by 33% (normal range not applicable).

d GI tract:
- gastro-oesophageal reflux 2nd and 3rd trimester and ± 48 h post-delivery therefore high risk of aspiration;
- constipation (increased gut transit time);
- raised alkaline phosphatase (liver).

68 When prescribing drugs to a pregnant patient the effects of the drug on the mother and fetus must always be considered. The earlier in the pregnancy that a drug is given, the greater the likelihood that it will cause a teratogenic problem. Drugs that are lipid-soluble, non-ionized and poorly protein-bound will cross the placenta. (As a rough rule of thumb, if a drug crosses the blood–brain barrier it will cross the placenta.) Always consult the British National Formulary (BNF) if in doubt about the effects of the drug.

Antibiotics, such as tetracycline and chloramphenicol, are contraindicated due to their effects on the fetal skeleton/dentition and bone marrow. Metronidazole is not contraindicated. All opioid analgesics will cross the placenta but should still be used if felt to be the most appropriate analgesic. This is only really a problem when delivery is imminent. Non-steroidal analgesics should be avoided if possible but paracetamol is safe.

C ☐
S ☐
R ☐

69   When managing the pregnant patient with surgical disease, it is important to:

- consider the well-being of the fetus;
- involve the obstetrician early;
- manage the patient with left lateral tilt/wedge to reduce aortocaval compression. Do not leave a heavily pregnant patient to lie flat on her back.

Peri-procedural management of steroids and immunosuppression

The physiological stress response to surgery and anaesthesia involves the release of catabolic hormones including catecholamines, human growth hormone, glucagon and corticosteroids. This response has implications for normal cardiovascular function in the face of this stress.

Therefore suppression of adrenocortical function by corticosteroid therapy for replacement or immunosuppression has important implications for surgical patients and must be carefully considered during the perioperative period to minimize risk to the patient.

In addition, other immunosuppressant drugs have important physiological effects, and their management around the time of surgery is also important.

Learning exercise	70

What are the most common reasons why a patient might be taking steroids or immunosuppressants?

Learning exercise	71

What are the equivalent anti-inflammatory doses of hydrocortisone, dexamethasone and triamcinolone for 10 mg of prednisolone?

Learning exercise	72

List the types of immunocompromised patients you might find in clinical practice.

Learning exercise	73

In the absence of a clear history, what clinical features and investigations suggest that a patient might be immunocompromised?

Learning exercise	74

What extra precautions will you take with these patients in the perioperative period?

Learning exercise	75

Name four unusual infective complications that you might be aware of when an immunocompromised patient presents with an as yet undiagnosed febrile episode.

See answers to learning exercises on page 159.

Try clinical case 12:

Clinical case 12

Karen Schmidt, a 35-year-old woman with rheumatoid arthritis, presents for open cholecystectomy. She took 10 mg of prednisolone/day until it was stopped 2 weeks ago.

Q1 How long after the commencement of therapy may the patient experience adrenal suppression?

Q2 Is 10 mg likely to suppress the endogenous response to surgery?

Q3 What are the main determinants of the dose of replacement steroid you would consider?

Clinical case 12 answers

Q1 Suppression may be seen after as little as 1 week of therapy while it may continue for as long as 3 months after stopping it.

Q2 While complete absence of hypothalamus–pituitary–adrenal axis (HPA) function (for example following adrenalectomy) prevents a normal response to surgery, it is not clear as to the clinical significance of reduced endogenous HPA function in those taking corticosteroids for immunosuppression; some evidence suggests no reduction in the response to surgery in those taking around 10 mg prednisolone/ day.

Q3 The doses of corticosteroid replacement therapy given during the perioperative period should reflect:

  ⌐ the duration of therapy;

  ⌐ the doses taken preoperatively;

  ⌐ the magnitude of the surgical stress.

The first two of these determine the extent of the HPA suppression, while the amount of glucocorticoid required to produce an adequate response to surgery depends on the third, whether the HPA is functioning well or not.

Answers to learning exercises

Periprocedural management of steroids and immunosuppression

70 The most common conditions for which a patient might be taking steroids or immunosuppressants are:

  ● asthma/chronic obstructive airways disease (COAD);

  ● rheumatoid arthritis;

  ● inflammatory bowel disease;

  ● vasculitis;

  ● cancer.

71 The anti-inflammatory doses equivalent to 10 mg prednisolone are:

  ● hydrocortisone 40 mg,

  ● dexamethasone 1.5 mg,

  ● triamcinolone 8 mg.

72 The types of immunocompromised patient that you might meet in clinical practice are:

- Congenital
  - Agammaglobulinaemia or hypogammaglobulinaemia.
- Acquired
  - Major trauma (including surgery) impairs immunity.
  - Blood dyscrasias—either diseases such as leukaemias or myelofibrosis or iatrogenic problems, such as drug-induced aplastic anaemia or splenectomy.
  - HIV.
  - Chemical immunosuppression with, for example steroids, azathioprine or cyclosporin A. The latter drug was an advance in that it was a more effective immunomodulator, suppressing humoral and cell-mediated immunity, and it proved to be less toxic to lymphoid tissue or bone marrow, but is nephrotoxic.
  - Medical diseases, such as diabetes, severe jaundice and renal disorders.
  - Advanced malignancy.
  - Blood transfusion is thought to be an adverse immunomodulator. Some data suggest that patients do not fare as well, for example patients with colonic carcinoma following excisional surgery for tumours, and therefore some caution is advised in giving a blood transfusion in such patients. There can be very few indications for giving a single unit transfusion to an adult.
  - Hypoxia.

73 In the absence of a history, other clues that a patient might be immunocompromised are:

- Unusual opportunistic infections, for example gastrointestinal infections, such as cryptosporidiosis, cytomegalovirus or giardiasis; respiratory infections, such as *Pneumocystis carinii*, *Legionella* or cytomegalovirus; skin infection with a fungus, mucormycosis or pyoderma gangrenosum; septicaemia from infections that would not usually cause septicaemia, for example an abscess or UTI.
- Low WCC.
- Specific tests of neutrophil function, for example measurement of neutrophil chemotaxis, or specific counts of different types of lymphocyte populations.

74 The extra precautions that you would take with these patients in the perioperative period are given below.

- Preoperative measures. In sick immunocompromised patients careful resuscitation is required, and senior anaesthetic and surgical staff need to be involved.
- Timing of operation. An appropriate, timely and simple operation is the ideal.
- Antibiotics. Sound antibiotic prophylaxis or therapy based on likely or proven bacterial contamination is of value and should be started as early as possible, certainly early enough to have high tissue levels at the start of operation.
- Operative technique. Minimize the extent of contamination and accumulation of haematomas, and perform gentle tissue dissection. Anastomoses should be avoided in an adverse environment (for example gross sepsis or ischaemia) but if carried out technique must be impeccable. Sepsis must be adequately drained, if

necessary leaving wounds widely open. There should be adequate clearance of contaminated fluids and tissues, and irrigation with fluid, either saline or tetracycline solution.

- Post-operative measures. Awareness of the possible sequelae of infection will mean that early diagnosis of problems may be made. Selective decontamination of the GI tract using antibiotics is of doubtful value.

75 Unusual infective complications that you might be aware of when the immunocompromised patient presents with a febrile episode are:

- Gastrointestinal infections, which usually present with diarrhoea and early intestinal perforation. These infections may be caused by *Cryptosporidium*, cytomegalovirus, *Salmonella* spp., *Shigella* spp., *Campylobacter jejuni*, *Giardia lamblia* and others.
- Respiratory infection caused by *Pneumocystis carinii*, *Legionella* or cytomegalovirus.
- Skin infections with a fungus, mucormycosis or pyoderma gangrenosum.
- Septicaemia may arise from infections that would not usually cause this problem, for example an abscess or a UTI.

Rheumatoid arthritis

This is a chronic disease, affecting not only the joints, but also most of the systems in the body. Of particular interest in the perioperative period is the effect rheumatoid arthritis, or its treatment, has on the:

- respiratory system;
- cardiovascular system;
- cervical spine;
- blood.

This section aims to outline the necessary features involved in the pre-assessment of a patient with rheumatoid arthritis.

Learning exercise	76

In terms of the skeletal systems, name the three joints that are of particular interest to the anaesthetist.

Learning exercise	77

a Concerning the C-spine, what radiographic position of the C-spine is most useful?

b What are the indications for X-radiography of the neck?

Learning exercise	78

Concerning the lung, what problems might there be with a patient with rheumatoid arthritis?

▼

What pulmonary investigations might you consider in assessing a patient with rheumatoid arthritis?

What are the cardiovascular problems associated with rheumatoid arthritis?

List the drugs that have been commonly used in the treatment of rheumatoid arthritis.

Many patients with rheumatoid arthritis wear cervical collars. What is your management of patients who do or do not wear collars?

Answers to learning exercises

76 In the patient with rheumatoid arthritis, the three joints that are of greatest interest to the anaesthetist are:

1 Cervical spine—instability occurs in 25% of patients with rheumatoid arthritis, with the commonest problem being atlanto-axial subluxation. Therefore, this might cause possible migration of the odontoid peg backwards and upwards, which may compress the spinal cord.

2 Temporomandibular joint—this is involved in ~80% of patients. This can cause reduced mouth opening, therefore making intubation difficult.

3 Cricoarytenoid joints—again this may make intubation difficult.

77 a The most useful radiographic position of the C-spine is a lateral and flexion X-ray. This will show the distance between the odontoid peg and the posterior border of the anterior arch of the atlas. With severe subluxation, fibreoptic intubation may be required.

b Patients with rheumatoid arthritis should have their necks X-rayed if they experience pain on neck movements or have a limited range of movement. This should be done prior to admission to allow experienced radiologists to assess the degree of subluxation, if present. Severe subluxation at C1/C2 presents a major hazard to the patient and will necessitate skilled anaesthetic presence.

78 A patient with rheumatoid arthritis might have any of the following problems relating to the lung:

- Pleural effusion—this occurs in ~10% of patients.
- Pulmonary nodules.
- Pulmonary fibrosis.
- Caplan's syndrome—nodular pulmonary fibrosis in a patient who has rheumatoid arthritis, and has been exposed to various industrial dusts.

▼

79   Pulmonary investigations that you might consider in assessing a patient with rheumatoid arthritis include:

- pulse oximetry;
- arterial blood gases;
- chest X-ray;
- spirometry and other pulmonary function tests—these depend on the clinical findings.

80   Cardiovascular problems associated with rheumatoid arthritis include:

- pericarditis;
- myocarditis;
- coronary arteritis causing myocardial ischaemia;
- conduction defects;
- pericardial effusion.

81   Drugs used in the treatment of rheumatoid arthritis include:

- paracetamol;
- NSAIDs;
- steroids;
- sulfasalazine (sulphasalazine);
- methotrexate;
- penicillamine;
- gold;
- immunosuppressants, such as azathioprine.

82   If a patient normally wears a collar then it is advisable to keep it on when the patient enters theatre. Anaesthesia will relax the muscles of the neck and will therefore reduce the support it will receive. If a patient does not normally wear a collar there seems little point in producing one for the operation.

Liver disease

C ☐
S ☐
R ☐

There may be a number of different guises in which the jaundiced patient presents. It may be via A & E, out-patients or the pre-admission clinic; they may present acutely with a medical or surgical cause, or they may have incidental disease coexisting with another surgical problem. The diagnosis and management of the jaundice is of paramount importance in these situations and we will briefly look at how the presence of jaundice and liver dysfunction as incidental findings affects the perioperative course of a patient presenting for elective surgery.

Many of the causes are not actually surgically related. However, it is still vital that you are aware of them as they may well have some bearing on the perioperative course of your patient. For example, an alcoholic patient may well suffer with delirium tremens during their admission or experience nutritional problems that may affect wound healing, infection, etc.

Learning exercise   83

What are the common causes of jaundice?

▼

Learning exercise	84

What aspects of the chronic liver disease will affect the course of your patient?

Learning exercise	85

How may ascites affect the perioperative course?

Learning exercise	86

How would you deal with a patient with large-volume ascites?

Learning exercise	87

What factors might induce a state of hepatic encephalopathy?

See answers to learning exercises on page 170.

Now try clinical cases 13 and 14:

Clinical case 13

Amy Williams, 26 year old, is admitted for elective surgery for a fibroadenoma. She has additionally suffered from arthralgia for 2 years and has been having menstrual irregularities with periods of amenorrhoea. She also suffered a bout of fever with cough and expectoration the previous week, which responded to a course of erythromycin. She is a non-smoker and a teetotaller. She is taking the oral contraceptive pill. On examination the only positive finding is a mild jaundice. When told of the finding, she says that her friends have, on three separate occasions, commented about her ocular yellowish discoloration since she suffered from hepatitis on returning from a holiday in Thailand 3 years ago. She had to be transfused following an accident there. Though she recovered quickly, the yellow tinge in her eyes persisted for 3 months.

Q1 What is your clinical impression of the case?

Q2 What additional history is needed?

Q3 What investigations would you ask for?

Q4 What would your management be?

Clinical case 13 answers

Q1 The most likely diagnosis is Gilbert's syndrome.

Recurrent episodes of jaundice in a young female could be due to:

- Gilbert's syndrome (asymptomatic mild jaundice which persisted following an episode of hepatitis in a young adult and recurrent deepening of jaundice under physical stress, fever, starvation, intercurrent infection, surgery and heavy alcohol ingestion).
- Drug-induced cholestatic hepatitis (on oral contraceptive pill, erythromycin).
- Chronic viral hepatitis B and C (HBV and HCV).
- Autoimmune hepatitis.

- Low-grade haemolytic disorders (mycoplasma pneumonia, systemic lupus erythematosus [SLE], secondary syphilis).
- Biliary parasites: *Clonorchis sinensis* and *Ascaris lumbricoides*.
- Others: acute ascending cholangitis, sclerosing cholangitis or early primary biliary cirrhosis are possible but unlikely here.

Q2   Additional features of her history needed are:

- whether she had noted a worsening of the jaundice on previous episodes with physical stress, fever, intercurrent infection, starvation and use of medicine;
- sexual promiscuity;
- intravenous drug use;
- Right upper quadrant (RUQ) pain, anorexia, nausea, vomiting;
- recent darkening of skin colour, unexpected persistence of a suntan;
- family history of jaundice;
- skin rash, photosensitivity.

Q3   You would request the following investigations:

- FBC, blood film examination for spherocytes, reticulocyte count, platelets.
- Prothrombin time (PT), INR, activated partial thromboplastin time (APTT).
- LFTs.
- Urea, creatinine, electrolytes.
- Serology for the viral hepatitis, especially HBsAg, IgM anti-HBc if HBsAg negative, HBe if HBsAg positive, anti-HCV.
- Serology for atypical pneumonia.
- Ultrasound of abdomen if predominantly conjugated hyperbilirubinaemia.

Q4   Demonstration of an increase in the bilirubin by >25 μmol/l after 2 days on a 300 kcal/day diet confirms the diagnosis of Gilbert's syndrome. The management should then be to:

- stop the drugs;
- make everybody concerned aware of the serology status;
- treat the aetiology.

 Clinical case 14

John Obeug, 62 years old, presents with upper abdominal pain and increasing jaundice.

Q1   Draw an appropriate algorithm of your plan of investigation.

Among the investigations was the ultrasound shown in Fig. 1.4.4.

Q2   Comment on the appearance of Fig. 1.4.4.

Fig. 1.4.4

Liver and biliary ultrasonogram

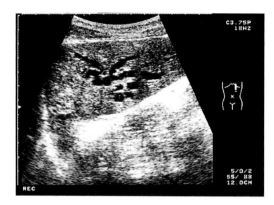

Q3 What precautions should you take in a jaundiced patient to prevent specific complications and why?

Clinical case 14 answers

Q1 An appropriate algorithm for the investigation of this patient is shown in Fig. 1.4.5.

Q2 The ultrasound scan shows dilated duct systems, both intrahepatic ducts and the common bile duct.

Q3 In a patient with jaundice the particular precautions that you can take to prevent complications are to:

- Check the fluid and electrolyte balance, ensure adequate urine output, give plenty of fluid and possibly 500 ml 20% mannitol to prevent acute tubular necrosis from the hepatorenal syndrome.

- Check prothrombin time (PT) and give 10 mg vitamin K_1 intravenously thrice daily until PT is normal, if you can wait for this. If not, fresh frozen plasma maybe required for immediate cover when the PT is >1.5.

- Give antibiotics either prophylactically or for established sepsis, for example a cephalosporin to prevent the greater risks from sepsis in such patients.

- Assess and correct nutritional status and serum albumin, particularly if there is associated malignancy or jaundice, to prevent problems with healing or from hypoalbuminaemia.

- Take great care with wound closure to prevent the increased tendency of wound failure in these patients.

- Possible early relief of jaundice, for example by stent, which reduces later surgical morbidity.

Fig. 1.4.5

Endoscopic retrograde cholangiopancreatography

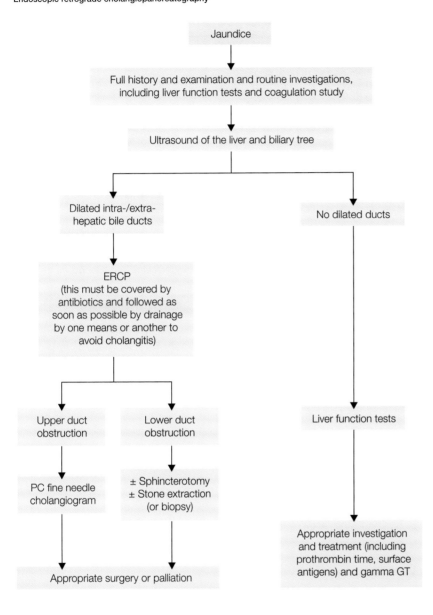

Renal failure

As with the jaundiced patient, you are going to encounter this associated condition in a number of different clinical situations. They can be placed in two broad categories:

1   The patient with chronic renal impairment presenting for surgery: renal or otherwise.
2   The patient with acute renal impairment either pre- or post-operatively.

It is unlikely that you will encounter true chronic renal failure without knowing of its existence. More likely you might find a mildly elevated urea and electrolytes on routine testing, and you must then know how to deal with these patients. Alternatively, an acute admission may have severely deranged results as a result of their acute condition.

The objectives of this section are:

- to know how to diagnose and manage uraemia in a new admission;
- to understand how to manage a patient with known established chronic renal failure.

Learning exercise	88

List the main causes of renal failure.

Learning exercise	89

How would you investigate a new admission with a urea of 50 mmol/l?

Learning exercise	90

Having established a diagnosis how would you then manage them?

Now we will cover how to deal with the patient who has chronic renal impairment who is presenting for surgery. What are their particular requirements and how do we deal with them? You will probably know that they can present with a variety of associated medical problems, each of which will require close observation and management.

Learning exercise	91

What aspects of care will you need to be aware of in a patient with interstitial nephritis and chronic renal impairment who is about to undergo major surgery?

See answers to learning exercises on page 170.

Think of the sort of operations that these patients might encounter. Obviously, they could require a number of procedures, but operations particularly associated with renal patients include:

- shunt insertion;
- dialysis line insertion;
- renal transplantation.

Obesity

You have looked at the impact of obesity on respiratory function earlier in this Unit. However, the obese patient presents many other problems and challenges for the surgeon. You should be thoroughly familiar with the risks of surgery and anaesthesia in the obese patient.

Learning exercise	92

List the possible complications in the obese patient:
a before surgery;
b during surgery;
c after surgery.

See answers to learning exercises on page 170.

Now try clinical case 15:

C ☐
S ☐
R ☐

Clinical case 15

Mrs Janet Tubbs, a 27-year-old mother of four, presents with an irreducible para-umbilical hernia. She weighs 22 stone and has been in pain, vomiting and had absolute constipation for 48 h.

Q1 What are the steps you would take in:

a Preparing her for theatre?

b Her post-operative management?

Clinical case 15 answer

Q1 a Preoperatively, you would take the following measures:

  ꓶ Informed consent should be obtained after explaining the nature of the problem to the patient.

  ꓶ Analgesia should be given as soon as the diagnosis is made and a course of action decided on.

  ꓶ The anaesthetist should see the patient, prior to theatre.

  ꓶ Put an intravenous line in the patient, and pass a nasogastric tube to keep the stomach empty, since she has intestinal obstruction secondary to the hernia.

  ꓶ Give subcutaneous heparin.

  ꓶ Investigations should include an FBC, urea and electrolytes, and a random blood sugar; also, serum should be sent for grouping.

  ꓶ If the periumbilical area is erythematous or has intertrigo, the region may be cleaned with povidone iodine, to help combat wound infection.

b Post-operatively, the following measures are taken:

  ꓶ Adequate analgesia may be given in the form of PCA, epidural analgesia, or intermittent intramuscular opiates, supplemented by infiltration of the wound by a longer-acting local analgesic, such as 0.5% bupivicaine (Marcain®) at the end of the operation.

  ꓶ There would be concern about hypoventilation after operation. Nurse the patient sitting up. Monitor the respiratory rate and check oxygen saturation. If there is concern check the blood gases.

  ꓶ Early mobilization is important, and regular observation of the wound should be undertaken to watch for bruising and infection.

Thyroid problems

You will remember from your undergraduate studies that the thyroid gland is an important contributor to the balance of metabolism. Consider the following learning exercise:

Learning exercise   93

Write out the clinical features of importance, risks and operative measures to be considered in a patient with thyroid disease about to undergo surgery.

See answers to learning exercises on page 170.

Answers to learning exercises

Liver disease

83   There are many causes of jaundice. Some of the more common causes are:

- haemolytic—increased rate of red cell destruction;
- hepatocellular—drugs, alcohol, viral hepatitis, congenital defects (Gilbert's disease, Crigler–Najjar syndrome, Dubin–Johnson syndrome);
- cholestatic—obstruction may be intrahepatic (drugs, alcohol) or extrahepatic (gallstones, tumour).

84   The following aspects of chronic liver disease might affect the course of your patient:

Fluid balance—Fluid management is difficult in patients with liver failure. The total body water and sodium is high and the total body potassium is low, due to secondary hyperaldosteronism despite intravascular hypovolaemia and hyponatraemia. Hypoalbuminaemia worsens peripheral oedema and ascites and predisposes to pulmonary oedema. Massive rapid fluid infusion bears the risk of rupture of the oesophageal varices. Large amounts of normal saline may precipitate pulmonary oedema and cause dilutional or rehydration acidosis.

Coagulopathy—Coagulation factors produced by the liver are I, II, V, VII, IX and X, of which II, VII, IX and X are vitamin K dependent. Factor VII has the shortest half-life and is lost first. Coagulopathy is due to:

- deficiency of vitamin K due to malabsorption of fat-soluble vitamins;
- impaired hepatic synthesis of the clotting factors;
- thrombocytopenia from hypersplenism, direct toxicity on the bone marrow of the toxin causing the chronic liver disease (alcohol, drugs, etc.).

Anaemia—This is due to:

- chronic GI blood loss from oesophageal varices, gastric erosions, piles;
- nutritional deficiencies (folate, B12, Fe);
- hypersplenism;
- toxic effects on the bone marrow;
- mild haemolysis due to acanthocytosis (spur-like projections on the red blood cell membrane due to deposition of cholesterol producing a membrane abnormality).

Metabolism of drugs

- drugs may worsen the liver failure;
- drugs are metabolized more slowly;
- levels of free drug (especially those that are highly protein-bound) in plasma due to hypoalbuminaemia.

Metabolic abnormalities

- hyperglycaemia due to insulin resistance, decreased hepatic glucose uptake, portosystemic glucose shunting and increased glucagon;
- hypoglycaemia due to reduced hepatic glucose synthesis, hepatic resistance to glucagon, poor oral intake, and hyperinsulinaemia due to portosystemic insulin shunting;

▼

- metabolic alkalosis due to hypokalaemia;
- respiratory alkalosis due to central hyperventilation in cirrhotics;
- hyperammonaemia;
- hypomagnesaemia, hypophosphataemia, hypocalcaemia;
- dilutional hyponatraemia;
- fat-soluble vitamin deficiencies.

85 Massive ascites produces several problems that might affect the perioperative course:

- mechanical pressure on the diaphragm impairs respiratory movement;
- increasing chances of basal atelectasis resulting in impaired gas exchange;
- overzealous attempts to treat it leads to haemodynamic and metabolic derangements;
- pressure over the renal vessels impairs renal perfusion with consequent impairment of renal function.

86 When managing a patient with large-volume ascites, large-volume paracentesis (4–6 litres) with appropriate fluid replacement during the procedure is safe when done with monitoring. Massive transfusion of normal saline produces dilutional or rehydration acidosis. Albumin and Ringer's solution are better options than normal saline. Lactated Ringer's solution is readily metabolized even in chronic liver failure.

87 The following factors might precipitate hepatic encephalopathy:

- excessive drainage of ascitic fluid without adequate volume replacement;
- overzealous use of diuretics in an attempt to reduce the oedema, producing intravascular hypovolaemia and hypokalaemic alkalosis;
- hypoxia;
- GI bleeding;
- excessive dietary protein to correct the hypoalbuminaemia;
- constipation;
- use of sedatives, narcotics;
- any systemic infection—manifest or occult, including spontaneous bacterial peritonitis (SBP);
- superimposed acute liver failure due to drugs and hepatic hypoperfusion.

Renal failure

88 The causes of renal failure can be divided into the following categories:

- Prerenal
  - dehydration;
  - haemorrhage;
  - sepsis;
  - burns;
  - CCF.
- Renal
  - glomerulonephritis;
  - vascular disease;
  - drugs, nephrotoxins;

- interstitial nephritis;
- myoglobinaemia;
- haemolysis.
- Postrenal
  - obstruction (prostate, tumour, stone).

89 Remember that many patients with a raised blood urea are dehydrated or have a mild degree of prostatic outflow obstruction and dehydration.

History

First you need a comprehensive history, asking in particular for:

- history of prostatism, diabetes, infection, previous renal disease;
- drug history—antibiotics (beta-lactams, aminoglycosides, amphotericin B), vasoconstrictors, NSAIDs, ACE inhibitors, diuretics, etc.;
- reasons for a low cardiac-output state which might lead to renal failure—for example diarrhoea and vomiting, gastrointestinal bleeding, burns, dehydration from acute abdomen, MI, CCF, etc.;
- examination should be directed towards these differential diagnoses.

Investigations

- Bloods—Hb, urea and electrolytes, creatinine level and creatinine clearance. Albumin levels indicate the degree of protein loss.
- Look at the urine for casts, WBC, blood and protein.
- Ultrasound of renal tracts to investigate possible dilation.
- Intravenous pyelogram (IVP).
- Renal biopsy may be indicated.

90 Depending on the cause, the management of renal failure would include referral to specialist urological or nephrology teams. Prerenal and postrenal causes should always be considered initially, and require prompt attention to prevent further renal damage.

Prerenal causes should be treated with rehydration against CVP measurement and the cause of the dehydration treated. For postrenal causes, the relief of obstruction is a priority—relieve urethral obstruction with a catheter or ureteric obstruction with stents or nephrostomies.

91 When caring for the surgical patient with interstitial nephritis you have to recall that many patients with chronic renal impairment are anaemic, are prone to acute renal failure, and can easily be overloaded with fluids. Drugs such as digoxin and gentamicin are excreted via the kidney and must be used with care, i.e. use a reduced dose initially and monitor the blood levels daily. Remember that patients with chronic renal failure can have hypercalcaemia, pericardial effusions, hyperkalaemia, fluid overload and malnutrition. Post-operative electrolyte disorders can occur, particularly hyponatraemia, acidosis, alkalosis and hypokalaemia. Care must be taken not to replace fluid losses with excessive amounts of isotonic or hypertonic saline solutions. This leads to hypernatraemia post-operatively, which can have a considerable mortality.

Obesity

92 Complications arising in the obese patient include:

a Before surgery:
   - Obese patients may pose problems in diagnosis. Abdominal tenderness may be less, with signs masked, and as a consequence, diagnosis of appendicitis or a perforated viscus may be delayed.
   - DVT not infrequently occurs preoperatively, partly from immobility.
   - Venous access is often limited.
   - There is an increased tendency in obese people to hypertension, diabetes, LVH, pulmonary hypertension, reflux arthritis and death.

b During surgery:
   - The patient may be heavy to move and lift.
   - Surgical access may be difficult, resulting in more complex operations of longer duration and larger incisions are needed.
   - Laparoscopic surgery is sometimes easier for patient and surgeon, but standard instruments may not be long enough.
   - There may be anaesthetic problems, particularly cardiovascular and respiratory. Monitoring may be unreliable.

c After surgery
   - Reduced mobility may lead to DVT, and exacerbation of arthritis.
   - Patients who are obese may be prone to chest complications, with atelectasis and hypercarbia, and it can be difficult to wean very obese people off the ventilator. Hypoventilation and obstructive sleep apnoea may compound this.
   - Wounds are more prone to haematomas, wound infection, wound dehiscence and incisional herniation.

Thyroid problems

93 The important clinical features, risks and perioperative precautions associated with thyroid disease are:

Clinical features

- goitre;
- stridor;
- tachycardia;
- occult myxoedema;
- clinical evidence of retrosternal extension;
- thyroid status.

Risks

- airway problems;
- difficult intubation;
- arrhythmias;
- bleeding;
- hypocalcaemia;
- RLN injury;

C ☐
S ☐
R ☐

- thyroid crisis.

Perioperative precautions

- bronchoscopic, bougie-guided intubation;
- propranolol;
- meticulous haemostasis;
- identify at least two parathyroid glands and both the nerves;
- prepare the patient with carbimazole or propyl thiouracil, or Lugol's iodine;
- (?Propranolol and/or sedative).

Clinical case 16

Daniel Lee, 56 year old, presents 24 h before his elective inguinal hernia repair. He gives a history of paroxysmal episodes of anxiety, flushing, palpitations, headaches and tremor. His BP readings vary, one noted to be as high as 230/120 mmHg and another one 140/90 mmHg. There are no other abnormal signs.

Q1   What is a possible diagnosis?

Q2   Are there any further investigations that may be useful?

Q3   What is the further management of this patient?

Q4   What are the other causes of secondary hypertension?

Q5   What are the complications of hypertension?

Clinical case 16 answers

Q1   These symptoms and signs may be caused by a phaeochromocytoma. If hypertension is found in the previously normal preoperative patient, then history and examination should be directed to eliciting possible causes of secondary hypertension, and in eliciting end-organ damage and cardiovascular complications.

Q2   Further investigations in this instance are urinary vanillylmandelic acid (VMA), computerized tomography (CT) / magnetic resonance imaging (MRI) of abdomen, etc. Again, special investigations directed towards possible causes or sequelae of hypertension will be suggested by the history and examination.

Q3   Often when a secondary cause of hypertension is suspected, surgery can be justifiably delayed to warrant further investigation and treatment. Phaeochromocytoma particularly should be excluded as this can cause life-threatening complications, the chances of which can be reduced with appropriate preoperative treatment.

Q4   Other secondary causes of hypertension include:
  - renal—chronic glomerulonephritis, chronic atrophic pyelonephritis, congenital polycystic kidneys, renal artery stenosis;
  - endocrine—Conn's syndrome, adrenal hyperplasia, phaeochromocytoma, Cushing's syndrome, acromegaly;
  - cardiovascular—coarctation of the aorta;
  - pregnancy;
  - drugs.

Q5 Complications of chronic hypertension include:
- ⊓ left ventricular hypertrophy;
- ⊓ myocardial ischaemia;
- ⊓ congestive cardiac failure;
- ⊓ aortic aneurysms;
- ⊓ renal impairment;
- ⊓ cerebral haemorrhages;
- ⊓ retinal changes.

C ☐
S ☐
R ☐

Radiology investigations

The Radiology department is an integral part of all acute hospitals, whether a large teaching institution or a small district general hospital. There is increasing awareness of the importance of timely, appropriate and accurate imaging in patient management and this has been coupled with huge expansion in imaging resources and equipment, although this expansion is currently lagging behind the increase in demand.

All radiology departments run differently and have differing sets of guidelines and protocols. It is important to become familiar with the local department—getting on well with radiographic and clerical staff is essential. It is also helpful to try and get to know the local consultant radiologists—learn who does what and when and also who is likely to help you out in a tight corner if you need something doing urgently.

Principles of utilizing the radiology department

Making a referral

Most radiologists regard a request for imaging as a clinical referral for an expert specialist opinion. Referrals are made using a request form and it is essential that these are filled out correctly, whether in paper or electronic format. Certain information is required including:

- patient identifier information (name, unit number, date of birth, etc.);
- in- or out-patient;
- ambulant, chair or bed;
- clinical history;
- investigation requested;
- form signed, dated, and requester contact details;
- other important information should also be included relating to renal function, diabetes, pregnancy, infection risk and allergy (which will be discussed later).

Always remember that if you are not sure which investigation you need discuss with the department, either radiographer or radiologist.

Prioritization

A department may receive hundreds of requests for all types of imaging each day. If you have a patient who needs an investigation urgently, try to discuss this in person—just writing 'urgent' on the form will not suffice. If a patient is particularly sick, let the radiographer know to minimize delays in the department.

Consent

Attitudes to consent have changed significantly over the previous few years. Informed patient consent means that a patient fully understands the benefits and risks of a procedure and is of sound mental state to make an informed judgement on these facts. As a doctor you should only obtain consent from a patient if you are fully conversant with the technique in question and ideally, certainly for invasive procedures, you should be able to perform the procedure. If you are unsure consult a senior colleague.

Verbal consent may suffice for certain radiological procedures that are relatively invasive, for example barium enema, contrast injection for intravenous urogram (IVU), with formal written consent needed for more invasive interventional procedures, for example angiography or biopsy—this is often performed by the performing radiologist.

Image interpretation

Interpretation of the image is usually undertaken by a radiologist or trained radiographer, and a formal report provided. Often initial image assessment, particularly of chest and abdominal X-rays is undertaken by more junior doctors. It is important that initial impressions of the radiographic image are documented in the patient notes, as always if unsure ensure a senior colleague has a look and document in the notes. The clinico-radiological meeting is an extremely useful forum for discussing difficult cases and obtaining advice for further imaging.

Audit/research

Many departments will be keen to assist or suggest topics suitable for audit and research. If you undertake an audit that involves radiology, liaise at the outset and confirm mechanisms for data collection and result dissemination on completion. Discuss research projects also, particularly if they involve additional ionizing radiation, as there are legal requirements around this and also issues over funding additional investigations. You should check with your Trust's Research and Development department in the first instance.

Patient safety within the radiology department

The use of ionizing radiation

Ionizing radiation is potentially hazardous, with the fetus particularly sensitive, especially in the first trimester, with risk of possible induction of carcinogenesis or fetal malformation. Many procedures in radiology involve ionizing radiation, often in high doses and a list of same more common investigations and associated dose is included in Table 18.

Table 18: Typical doses from diagnostic medical exposure. (Modified from Royal College of Radiologists handbook, Making the Best Use of the Radiology Department, 5th edn.)

Diagnostic procedure	Typical effective dose (mSv)	Equivalent number of chest X-rays	Approximate equivalent period of natural background radiation
Radiographic examinations:			
Limbs and joints (except hip)	<0.01	<0.5	<1.5 days
Chest (single PA film)	0.02	1	3 days
Skull	0.06	3	9 days

Diagnostic procedure	Typical effective dose (mSv)	Equivalent number of chest X-rays	Approximate equivalent period of natural background radiation
Thoracic spine	0.7	35	4 months
Lumbar spine	1.0	50	5 months
Hip	0.4	20	2 months
Pelvis	0.7	35	4 months
Abdomen	0.7	35	4 months
IVU	2.4	120	14 months
Barium swallow	1.5	75	8 months
Barium meal	2.6	130	1 5 months
Barium follow-through	3	150	16 months
Barium enema	7.2	360	3.2 years
CT head	2.0	100	10 months
CT chest	8	400	3.6 years
CT abdomen or pelvis	10	500	4.5 years
Radionuclide studies:			
Lung ventilation (Xe-133)	0.3	15	7 weeks
Lung perfusion (Tc-99m)	1	50	6 months
Bone (Tc-99m)	4	200	1.8 years

Abbreviations: CT—computed tomography; IVU—intravenous urogram; PA—posteroanterior; UK average background radiation = 2.2 mSv per year; regional averages range from 1.5 to 7.5 mSv per year.

There are rules and regulations controlling the use of ionizing radiation documented in the ionizing radiation (medical exposure) regulations, published in 2000 (IRMER) and these are legally binding. Certain principles will help you use X-rays more safely:

- Do no harm. Does the patient need the X-ray? Could another investigation be used more safely that does not involve ionizing radiation, for example ultrasound or magnetic resonance imaging.
- Has the test already been done? Check patient notes—do not request serial chest or abdominal X-rays or in chronically sick patients, unless you feel patient management will be affected.
- Is the timing correct? It is difficult to analyse poor quality radiographs—it may sometimes be better to allow acute symptoms to settle to optimize imaging parameters.
- Has the most appropriate investigation been requested? If not sure discuss.

Patient identification and confidentiality

Problems with patient identification are common—correct provision of patient details to radiology, usually on the request form, is extremely important to prevent these. As in all other areas, avoid discussing patient details or results where confidentiality may be compromised.

Pregnancy

As previously mentioned, the fetus must be protected from the effects of ionizing radiation wherever possible. Departments will have protocols for the use of X-rays in pregnancy. For repeat exposures investigations, for example IVU and barium enema, the test should be done within ten days of the first day of the last period (the 'ten-day rule')— this extends to 28 days for a single exposure only of chest X-ray. In all cases the patient needs to sign a disclaimer that they are not pregnant prior to exposure. If in any doubt do a pregnancy test.

In an emergency, for example computed tomography in trauma, the clinical need may override safety concerns, but efforts will be made to shield the fetus (lead shielding, etc.). Record all decisions in patient notes.

Always ensure that you have excluded pregnancy and a disclaimer is signed before patients go to theatre where ionizing radiation is to be used, for example image intensifier in orthopaedic procedure or for operative cholangiography, both of which are common in women of child-bearing age. If the disclaimer has not been signed, the patient will have to be woken from anaesthetic and sign the form once anaesthetic has worn off.

Allergy and asthma

Many contrast agents contain iodine and the department should be informed if a patient has a history of iodine hypersensitivity. Minor reactions to iodine are not uncommon (rash, wheeze) with severe anaphylaxis (1 in 1000) and death (1 in 12 000–40 000) relatively rare. In those with a history of contrast reaction, or at high risk (including asthmatics) consider pre-medication with steroids, or another investigation—these decisions should be made in liaison with radiology.

Renal impairment and diabetes

Intravenous, iodine-based, contrast agents are potentially nephrotoxic with increased risk in renal impairment, diabetes mellitus, dehydration, myeloma and the elderly. Contrast agents should be avoided in the at-risk and liaison with radiology is again important.

Many diabetics are on treatment with oral metformin and these patients are at risk of lactic acidosis and renal failure following intravenous contrast administration. Metformin should be stopped on the day of the test and for 48 hours post-injection and serum urea and electrolytes should be monitored if impaired pre-procedure.

Infection

Patients and staff within the radiology department expect to be protected from possible cross-infection. For this to occur, patients with communicable infections must be identified to the department before they come for their investigation to allow protection measures to be taken. Infections to be notified would include MRSA, HIV, hepatitis, tuberculosis, infective diarrhoea, for example *Clostridium difficile*, *Escherichia coli*. Remember that an MRSA patient may need to be placed at the end of a list, just as in theatre, to facilitate adequate cleansing of the room.

Imaging modalities

This section of the unit deals with the major imaging modalities in outline. It is not intended to be fully comprehensive but to act as an overview for each technique. Your Trust may subscribe to the The Royal College of Radiologists' publication *Making the best use of a department of clinical radiology: guidelines for doctors*, which does provide a good overall guide to investigation types and indications.

Conventional X-rays (radiographs, plain film)

In many departments conventional radiography is being replaced by digital radiography where the X-ray film is replaced by a digital screen. This digital information can be manipulated by computers and the image visualized on a monitor—the department is 'filmless'. Images can be stored and viewed using PACS (picture archiving and communication system). Although expensive and potentially catastrophic if they break-down, these systems offer advantages of:

- decreased radiation dose;
- improved image quality;
- reduced storage problems;
- no lost films;
- ease of availability of films and reports for clinicians.

The chest X-ray

Along with the abdominal X-ray, the chest X-ray probably represents the most commonly requested investigation by the junior doctor. This is coupled with the fact that these radiographs are often difficult to interpret and initial interpretation is often made by a junior doctor faced with a sick patient in the middle of the night! Tailor the timing of the radiograph according to the clinical need—can the chest X-ray wait till the morning?

The chest X-ray is relatively low dose, but this dose can accumulate rapidly (as with abdominal X-ray) if serial tests are performed.

Indications

Usually there are many indications, but always justify the exposure—will it change your management? Indications might include, as one or in combination:

- shortness of breath;
- chest pain—pleuritic or non-pleuritic;
- haemoptysis;
- cough—dry/productive;
- wheezing.

Chest X-rays should not be performed preoperatively on a routine basis. Departments will have protocols: acute chest symptoms/signs or worsening of pre-existing chest condition would require imaging.

Views

- PA (postero-anterior)—X-ray beam passes from back to front of patient during full inspiration. The ideal routine projection and allows evaluation of heart size (the CTR-cardiothoracic ratio [see Fig. 1.4.6]). PA films do require the patient to be mobile and able to stand and are often not feasible in the acutely unwell.

- AP (antero-posterior) with X-ray beam passing from front to back. This view magnifies the heart-size (further from film) and usually precludes accurate evaluation of cardiomegaly or mediastinal contour. AP films are often the only view possible acutely and can be taken with the patient sat up in bed, with the film behind them. Views are often of poor quality and follow-up films in the department may be needed.
- Lateral views are less widely used. Generally discuss with the radiologist before requesting this.
- Apical/lordotic projections may occasionally be recommended for upper zone lesions.

The normal chest X-ray

Check for gross abnormality and then specific review areas. Check:

- patient name, date of film, film markers (right and left);
- degree of inspiration, penetration, rotation and projection (AP or PA);
- heart size (if PA);
- mediastinal contour? Widened (mediastinal haematoma) hilar mass or displacement;
- lungs;
- bones;
- soft tissues;
- review areas, i.e. those sites where lesions may be missed for example beneath diaphragm, behind heart, lung apices.

The abnormal chest X-ray

Clearly a wide range of pathology may be manifest on a chest X-ray, well beyond the scope of this text. What may you see on a chest X-ray?

- Cardiomegaly and evidence of cardiac failure, for example pleural effusions, lung infiltrates or airspace oedema.
- Evidence of consolidation of whatever cause.
- Focal or multiple lung lesions. There is a broad differential diagnosis for these appearances, although malignancy should always be considered.
- Evidence of perforation of an abdominal viscus with sub-diaphragmatic free air—this may be miniscule or massive. Interposed bowel between liver and diaphragm (Chilaiditi's syndrome) may mimic free air.

Learning exercise	94

a   What abnormalities can you see on Figures 1.4.6, 1.4.7, 1.4.8? Use the arrows as a guide.

b   What do the measurements A and B indicate in Fig. 1.4.6 and how can they be used?

Fig. 1.4.6

Courtesy of Eastbourne District General Hospital, East Sussex

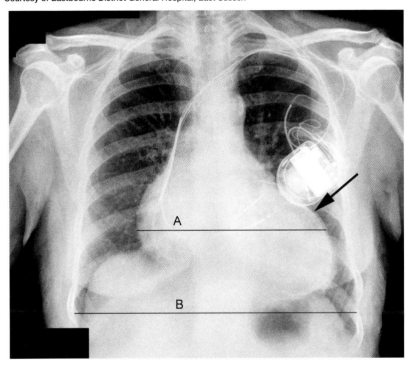

Fig. 1.4.7

Courtesy of Eastbourne District General Hospital, East Sussex

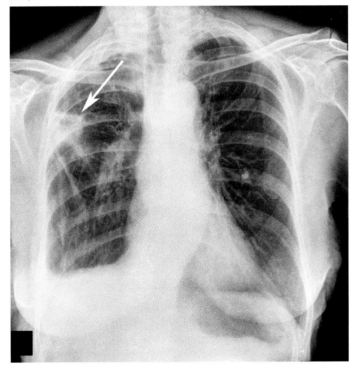

Fig. 1.4.8

Courtesy of Eastbourne District General Hospital, East Sussex

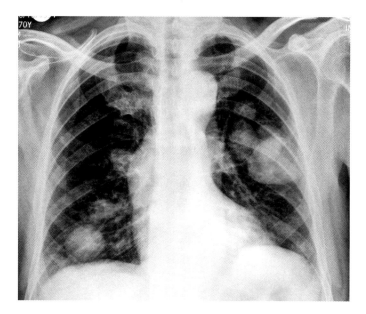

Answers to learning exercise

94 Fig. 1.4.6 PA chest X-ray to demonstrate cardiomegaly. The cardio-thoracic ratio (CTR) is measured using maximum cardiac measurement (line A) divided by maximum intrathoracic measurements (line B) and if greater than 50% in an adult; as in this case, this is indicative of cardiomegaly. This patient also has a dual-lead pacemaker in-situ and note curvilinear calcification projected over the left ventricular apex (arrow)—this relates to a calcified left ventricular aneurysm, probably post-previous MI.

Fig. 1.4.7 PA chest X-ray demonstrates a peripheral opacity in the right mid-zone which contains central lucency secondary to cavitation (arrow). This lesion is a primary squamous cell carcinoma. Fibrotic charges are present in the right lung and a right basal pleural effusion is also present.

Fig. 1.4.8 PA chest X-ray demonstrates multiple lung metastases secondary to renal cell carcinoma.

Contrast studies

Barium studies

Barium sulphate is an insert contrast agent used to opacify the gastrointestinal tract. It comes in a variety of suspensions designed for specific purposes—it is important when requesting a barium study to be clear what area is to be assessed as this will affect suspension used and patient preparation. Discuss with the department if unsure.

Types of barium study include:

- barium swallow;
- barium meal—less used now as endoscopy is technique of choice for initial assessment of the stomach and oesophagus;

C ☐
S ☐
R ☐

▼

- small bowel follow through/enema—used for small bowel evaluation. The small bowel enema is invasive requiring passage of a nasojejunal tube, which may not be well tolerated and also entails a high radiation dose.
- barium enema.

Points to remember:

- Barium is contraindicated in suspected bowel perforation (causes a mediastinitis or peritonitis). In these cases consider a water-soluble contrast agent—discuss with department.
- Barium enema is contraindicated if deep rectal biopsy is performed within the previous 5 days.
- Barium enema requires formal large bowel preparation with laxatives. The elderly or infirm may need to be admitted for this and laxatives are contraindicated in the presence of suspected obstruction.
- Barium causes artefact on CT making it hard to interpret for up to 2 weeks.

Non-ionic agents are more expensive, but safer and are used for intravenous and intra-arterial injections, for example IVU, computed tomography, angiography and also in children.

Learning exercise 95

Figures 1.4.9–1.4.10 are examples of contrast studies. What are they and what do they indicate?

Fig. 1.4.9

Courtesy of Eastbourne District General Hospital, East Sussex

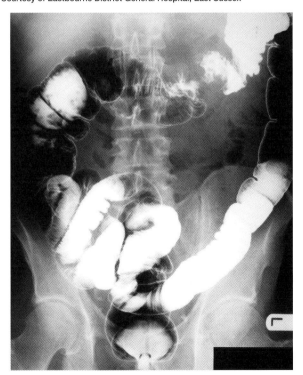

Fig. 1.4.10

Courtesy of Eastbourne District General Hospital, East Sussex

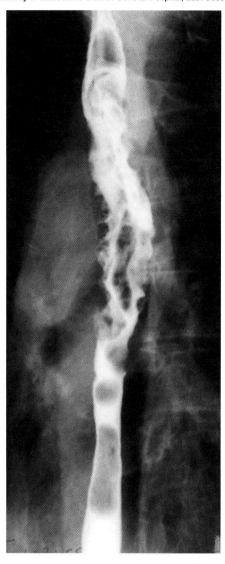

Answers to learning exercises

95   Fig. 1.4.9 Film from a double contrast barium enema shows an 'applecore' stricture in the left transverse colon consistent with a carcinoma.

Fig.1.4.10 Barium swallow study showing an extensive oesophageal carcinoma.

Ultrasonography (Ultrasound)

Ultrasound uses high-frequency sound waves generated from a transducer, which penetrate tissues and are reflected back. An image is created depending on how much sound is received by the transducer. Objects appear as black (hypoechoic) if they transmit sound well, reflecting little back, for example water, or as white (hyperechoic) if highly reflective such as gallstones. Colour Doppler ultrasound is a useful adjunct used to examine moving structures using the Doppler principle of a shift in sound frequency from moving structures to assess flow velocity and direction.

Uses of ultrasonography include:

- Abdomen/pelvis and chest. FAST (focused assessment for the sonographic examination of the trauma patient) scanning is used in some centres for rapid evaluation of the abdomen, in trauma patients, looking mainly for fluid.
- Breast, soft tissues, thyroid, tendons, testis.
- Vascular—arteries, veins, cardiac.
- Obstetrics.
- Neonatal brain, abdomen, hip.
- Endoscopic—upper and lower gastrointestinal tract. Different probes are available to improve visualization, for example transrectal (prostate, rectum), transvaginal, endoscopic (upper and lower gastro-intestinal tract).

Advantages of ultrasonography include:

- inexpensive;
- safe—no ionizing radiation;
- portable and can image in any plane;
- can guide biopsy/drainage procedures.

Disadvantages of ultrasonography are:

- highly operator dependent;
- highly patient dependent—utility of ultrasound in the abdomen is significantly degraded by bowel gas and adipose tissue and also by bone.

| Learning exercise | 96 |

Look at Figures 1.4.11 and 1.4.12. What do these examinations show (NB: The arrows may assist you!)?

Fig. 1.4.11

Courtesy of Eastbourne District General Hospital, East Sussex

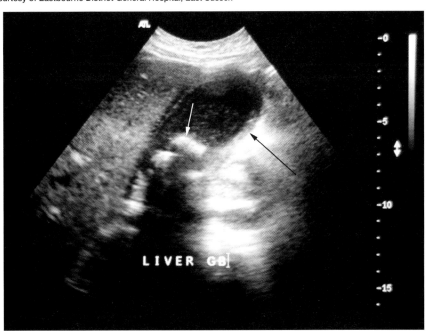

Fig. 1.4.12

Courtesy of Eastbourne District General Hospital, East Sussex

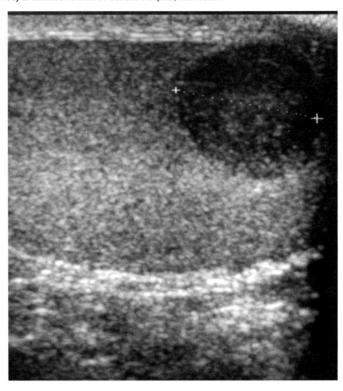

C ☐
S ☐
R ☐

Answers to learning exercise

96   Fig. 1.4.11 Sonogram of the gallbladder in acute cholecystitis. The gallbladder is thick-walled (black arrow) and contains internal calculi (white arrow) and sludge.

Fig. 1.4.12 Sonogram of the testis in a patient with a seminoma—note the hypoechoic, circumscribed mass at lower pole (callipers).

Sedation

As we have seen, many patients having minor, or even major, surgery do not necessarily require general anaesthesia. Indeed, in Scandinavian countries some 50% of operations are performed without general anaesthesia. However, even though they may not feel any pain or discomfort, the addition of sedation to an local anaesthetic technique helps remove some of the fear and concern that patients may have, and it acts as a useful adjunct to the local anaesthetic. In addition, many patients prefer to be sedated during GI endoscopy or bronchoscopy.

It is important for every doctor to consider what might go wrong when a patient is sedated and how to deal with it.

In this section, we will cover:

- drugs available for sedation;
- techniques for sedation;
- patient management during sedation;
- patient selection for sedation.

▼

Let's explore the ideas that have been introduced here a little further. You will all administer sedation at some time and you must be safe and confident in its use. Many people regard it as safe because it avoids general anaesthesia. However, if used incorrectly it has the potential for disaster—especially when you are the sole practitioner.

The main aim of this section is to ensure you apply the basic principles to your own practice and that you are, above all else, safe.

You may well know that there are a number of drugs which are commonly used today. Midazolam is the drug of choice because it has a short duration of action with a clear-headed recovery and has no active metabolite that may cause a hangover effect. Being water-soluble it is not thrombophlebitic. Also it can be reversed easily (learning exercise 102). Diazepam is the other benzodiazepine which might be used but it has a much longer duration of action and is not so easily reversed.

Not all patients are suited to receive sedation. The list of patients 'at risk' during sedation is long but includes:

- children;
- the elderly;
- the morbidly obese;
- hypovolaemia—those with acute gastrointestinal bleeding are most at risk;
- coexistent cardiorespiratory disease is, of course, cause for concern;
- decreased level of consciousness.

Precautions to be taken before administering sedation are:

- oxygen;
- suction;
- resuscitation drugs;
- tipping trolley;
- help is close at hand;
- intravenous access.

Drugs added to sedatives are:

Opiates such as morphine, pethidine or fentanyl.

Beware:

- adds to sedative effect;
- reduces ventilation;
- CVS depression.

ALWAYS carefully titrate dose of drugs against response.

Learning exercise	97

How would you define sedation and how does it differ from general anaesthesia?

Learning exercise	98

List four advantages of sedation.

Learning exercise   99

List three disadvantages of sedation.

Learning exercise   100

Is intravenous administration the only route we can use? Why?

Learning exercise   101

What precautions should be observed for a patient before an upper GI endoscopy commences.

Learning exercise   102

What three monitors are mandatory during sedative procedures? How long would you continue to monitor your patient after the procedure?

Learning exercise   103

What instructions are you going to give the patient who has received sedation as a day case?

Learning exercise   104

What is the major problem of adding opiates to the sedative mixture?

Learning exercise   105

How can we reverse the effects of these drugs and what are the limitations of such reversal?

This section should have clarified a number of points and led you to think more about how sedation should be administered safely.

Sedation is potentially dangerous and should not be undertaken lightly or without the correct preparation.

Answers to learning exercises

97   Sedation involves the administration of drugs to alleviate patient discomfort and distress during diagnostic and therapeutic interventions. The patient must be able to respond to commands and communicate with the operator and thus will maintain protective reflexes. General anaesthesia renders the patient unconscious and abolishes these reflexes, so it is important to carefully titrate the drug to effect during sedation to avoid overdose.

98   The four advantages of sedation are:

1   amnesia for the procedure;

2   rapid recovery and minimal hangover—if the correct drugs are used appropriately;

3   maintenance of reflexes;

4   avoidance of general anaesthesia—by retaining patient communication, sedation

has considerable benefits. In addition, it obviates the need for the presence of an anaesthetist in every case, provided adequate precautions are observed.

99 Three disadvantages of sedation are given below.

1 Potential for overdose—the individual response to a drug is very variable. The conflicting demands of the operator needing good conditions for the procedure and of the patient needing to be comfortable can easily result in too much being given.

2 Failure to detect impending problems—particularly with a sole operator.

3 Minimal effect on pain—though may be combined with opiates (beware!).

100 No, it isn't. The oral and rectal routes have the disadvantage of unpredictable absorption and hence unpredictable effects. Inhalational sedation with entonox, which is really an analgesic, is useful both in terms of safety and speed of onset/offset.

101 The precautions are:

- check that oxygen, suction, resuscitation equipment and drugs are immediately available;
- check (by yourself) that such equipment is working;
- check that the table or trolley being used can be tipped head down;
- ensure that adequate help, i.e. another suitably trained individual, is present;
- obtain intravenous access using an indwelling cannula.

102 Minimal monitoring should include ECG, pulse oximeter and non-invasive blood pressure recording. ECG will give information on heart rate and rhythm but is not an indicator of adequate perfusion. A low oxygen saturation may reflect a poor cardiac output and if the oximeter probe is not reading do not assume it has fallen off—it may be unable to detect a pulse.

Monitor patients after the procedure until return of consciousness and all cardiorespiratory parameters have returned to normal levels.

103 Instructions to the patient include:

- They must be accompanied home by a responsible adult with written instruction on who to contact and what to do in the event of problems.
- They must not drive or operate machinery, nor sign legally binding agreements for 24 h.

104 When adding opiates to the sedative mixture, it is very easy to run into problems of oversedation and profound respiratory and/or cardiovascular depression. Modification of drug dose is essential. It is recommended that the opioid is given first and its effects carefully monitored before giving the benzodiazepine.

105 Naloxone (Narcan) can be given to reverse opiate drugs, and flumazenil is a specific benzodiazepine antagonist. The limitations are mainly related to duration of action of the antagonist, which is short and will soon wear off, leading to the risk of re-sedation occurring later. Reversal of overdose does not exclude the necessity for airway management and oxygenation, and close observation throughout recovery.

C ☐
S ☐
R ☐

Principles of anaesthesia

What is anaesthesia? At its simplest level an anaesthetic consists of the three components of unconsciousness, analgesia and muscle relaxation, which are produced in a controlled manner so that the patient has no recall of the procedure and the surgeon has the benefit of good operating conditions.

Traditionally anaesthesia has been divided into stages of induction, maintenance and recovery. While this is true of the perioperative period, the anaesthetist is now so heavily involved in both the preoperative assessment and the post-operative monitoring and management that these stages must also be included in describing the anaesthetist's role.

Nowadays, the anaesthetist has become much more involved in the pre-and post-operative care of the patient

The principal reason for this is that we are faced with the challenge of more elderly patients, many with coexistent medical disorders, who require increasingly complex surgery. The anaesthetist must be aware of patients' physiological reserve and their ability to cope with the stress of surgery, particularly in the post-operative period. The anaesthetist is intimately involved with the reaction of the patient to the stress of surgery and anaesthesia, and needs to be able to predict any eventuality.

In this section we are going to look at:

- important aspects of preoperative preparation;
- premedication;
- how anaesthesia is performed;
- some of the common drugs used by anaesthetists;
- monitoring.

Earlier in this Unit, you were introduced to many of the medical conditions that might be of concern to the anaesthetist. As we shall see, the most important aspect of the preoperative assessment is deciding whether the patient has a long-term medical condition which is under control (in which case delay or adjustment of treatment is probably unnecessary) or whether any medical problem is acute or an acute exacerbation of a chronic condition. In this situation you should seek the advice of the anaesthetist about how to proceed and what end-points to achieve which would ensure a safe progress through surgery.

Let us now review this by looking at how we can identify some of the more common problems. The three important areas of the preoperative assessment of the patient are taking a history, examining the patient and ordering the most relevant investigations.

The first aspect of assessment is history taking.

Learning exercise	106
In questioning a patient over 60 years old, name three important symptoms that would indicate cardiac disease and three important symptoms that would indicate respiratory disease.	

Learning exercise 107

Name three conditions that could predispose to cardiac disease that you would seek to identify in your history taking.

Learning exercise 108

Asthma is increasingly common in the population. In obtaining a history from an asthmatic patient, what do you think are the five most important elements?

Learning exercise 109

You will ask patients about allergies to drugs and many will give you long lists of drugs which upset them. What key elements will help to identify a true allergy?

Learning exercise 110

Apart from the cardiorespiratory disorders can you name four medical conditions that would cause the anaesthetist concern?

Let us have a quick look at some important aspects of the examination:

Learning exercise 111

List three important signs of cardiac failure.

Learning exercise 112

What level of hypertension is likely to be of concern to the anaesthetist and what factors are important when checking a patient's blood pressure?

Learning exercise 113

A 62-year-old male patient has a 10-year history of angina. Will his preoperative ECG show signs of myocardial ischaemia? Why?

Learning exercise 114

A 36-year-old woman is admitted for varicose vein surgery. She is a well-controlled asthmatic who takes a Becotide inhaler daily and salbutamol inhaler when required.
a   Should she have a chest X-ray preoperatively? Why?
b   Should she have an FBC? Why?

See answers to learning exercises on page 192.

It is obviously important to identify those patients at the risk of developing problems during or after surgery, particularly those undergoing elective procedures as it may be possible to delay surgery to optimize their condition. As we discussed earlier, a number of principles relating to the medical condition must be considered preoperatively when assessing the fitness for anaesthesia and surgery:

1   **Chronic disease.** We often have to accept that patients are not great physical specimens and are suffering from long-term conditions that may have an influence on

▼

their outcome. The important aspect of this is to ensure that:

- they are in as good shape as they can be despite their medical problems;
- the anaesthetist is aware of potential problems well in advance of surgery so that all the necessary arrangements can be made (for example ITU available, consultant cover, etc.) and a management plan drawn up (cancelling operations at the last minute often turns out to have been avoidable);
- the anaesthetic technique can be planned in advance.

2 **Acute disease.** Acute changes in medical condition need to be treated/controlled prior to surgery. This obviously depends on the nature of the surgery:

- elective surgery—should be postponed so that the necessary treatment can be instituted (for example chest infection, tachyarrhythmia);
- emergency surgery—frequently the medical derangement may be the result of the surgical condition. Whatever, it is a judgement call on the day how far to go with resuscitation and treatment at the expense of a worsening surgical or medical condition.

Whenever patients are seen preoperatively, they can be graded according to the risk of undergoing surgery. This largely relates to the medical condition of the patient and the type of surgery planned for them. While for many patients the risk is relatively low compared with the benefits of surgery, there are some in whom considerable risk is attached to proceeding without conferring much perceived benefit. The main risk classification systems are the ASA grade (covered previously in this unit) and the more complex Goldman classification.

It is this risk stratification that helps the anaesthetist guide his decision as to when, or if to anaesthetize a patient for surgery. So, next time you are preparing a list, or more importantly admitting patients on call, try to grade them using these systems. These classifications do not pretend to provide all the answers as to whether to proceed to surgery, but they do help in pointing us towards a decision.

Answers to learning exercises

106 The most important symptoms of cardiac disease and respiratory disease are:

- cardiac disease—angina, shortness of breath, palpitations, syncope;
- respiratory disease—shortness of breath, wheeze, cough and sputum production;
- as you can see breathlessness can be the result of both cardiac or lung disease, and further questioning and investigations will be required to differentiate between them. Orthopnoea and paroxysmal nocturnal dyspnoea are usually indicators of cardiac rather than respiratory disease, while exercise tolerance is a good indicator of cardiorespiratory reserve.

107 The main predisposing conditions for cardiac disease are hypertension, diabetes, smoking, obesity and hypercholesterolaemia.

108 Important elements to obtain in a history from an asthmatic patient are:

- what their best peak flow measurement is;
- frequency of attacks is an important feature of the severity of the asthma;
- history of hospitalization to control an attack;
- medication taken by the patient is also a helpful indicator and in particular the need

for systemic steroid therapy (prednisolone), which would suggest more significant disease;

- many asthmatics have a seasonal variability in their symptoms so the timing of surgery may be influenced by this.

109   A history of swelling around the face and mouth in association with blotches or redness of the skin is much more indicative of a true allergic response than symptoms of gastrointestinal upset, which can occur with any drug.

110   The list of medical conditions that would cause the anaesthetist's concern is endless. However, diabetes, renal failure, rheumatoid arthritis and any neuromuscular disorder are associated with a significant risk of perioperative anaesthetic problems and the anaesthetist would wish to assess these patients carefully.

111   Cardiac failure is basically a failure of the pump function of the heart resulting in an inability to provide the cardiac output and oxygen delivery requirements of the body. It may affect the left ventricle, the right ventricle or on occasions there is biventricular (congestive) failure. The signs depend on which ventricle is affected. If it is left ventricular failure, this produces pulmonary oedema and the clinical signs of:

1   basal crepitations, tachycardia and gallop rhythm with a third heart sound and dyspnoea and orthopnoea.

2   If right ventricular failure occurs either as a consequence of prolonged pulmonary hypertension secondary to hypoxia, as in chronic obstructive airways disease, or as a result of chronic severe left ventricular failure, this produces:

3   ankle oedema, hepatomegaly and raised jugular venous pressure.

112   A diastolic BP above 110 mmHg is generally as high as most anaesthetists would accept. The reasons for concern are that untreated hypertension such as this is associated with significant and often frightening swings in blood pressure during the perioperative period which can result in MI or stroke. It should be treated before surgery whenever possible. The size of the cuff can have a big influence on the reading obtained as too small a cuff may result in an abnormally high reading. The cuff width/arm circumference ratio should be 0.4–0.6 to avoid errors.

113   No, not necessarily. A resting ECG in many cases will not demonstrate any sign of ischaemia. Stress testing will be more likely to indicate the problem or alternatively the use of 24 h ECG recording. Unfortunately, these are difficult to perform and the number of patients is large.

114   The answers are:

a   No. In the absence of specific respiratory symptoms, a chest X-ray is of limited value.

b   An FBC is not indicated for the above patient.

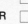

C ☐
S ☐
R ☐

Process of general anaesthesia

We are now at the stage where we should have a reasonable understanding of the processes involved in the anaesthetic work-up of the patient prior to theatre, and the amount of risk they are due to undertake for the privilege.

Let us now move on to the process of giving an anaesthetic, where we shall look at some of the drugs anaesthetists use, why they use them and the effects – good and bad – of their use.

The process of anaesthesia is basically split into three parts:

1   Induction, where the patient is rendered unconscious prior to commencing of surgery. This may be achieved either by using intravenous agents or inhalational agents. The intravenous route is generally quicker and simpler but does involve an intravenous cannula, which can be distressing, particularly for children.

2   Maintenance, where we keep the patient asleep either by continuing with the intravenous agent as an infusion or where we continue to administer inhalational agent throughout the case. As we have discussed, modern anaesthesia consists of a number of different drugs, and we may use analgesics (usually opioids) and muscle relaxants to augment the basic hypnotic anaesthetic drugs.

3   Recovery, where we reduce the concentration of anaesthetic we are giving so that the patient is allowed to wake up slowly, and we reverse the effects of the muscle relaxants.

One of the effects of anaesthesia and muscle relaxation is hypotension. This is one of the major considerations for anaesthetists in their choice of induction agent, particularly in the emergency situation.

You will have frequently encountered emergencies where you want to proceed into theatre as quickly as possible only to encounter delay from your anaesthetic colleague. This is usually time well spent. Many emergency patients are profoundly fluid-depleted intravascularly and only maintaining their BP by vasoconstriction and tachycardia. If we were now to abolish this constriction with our anaesthetic agents we would induce a catastrophic fall in BP and possibly arrest. These patients must be rehydrated before surgery.

Learning exercise	115

Name the most commonly used induction agents. What factors are taken into consideration when choosing between them?

Learning exercise	116

Other than CNS depression, name two other major organ systems affected by general anaesthetics and what these effects are.

Learning exercise	117

In what situations may these effects be more pronounced?

▼

| Learning exercise | 118 |

What is the importance of adequate preoperative resuscitation?

| Learning exercise | 119 |

What methods are available to control the airway?

| Learning exercise | 120 |

Why does the anaesthetist use muscle relaxants?

| Learning exercise | 121 |

What are the principal differences between an laryngeal mask airway (LMA) and intubating a patient?

See answers to learning exercises on page 198.

In addition, during such emergencies where fluid balance is in question we will frequently use intravascular monitoring to guide us. This will certainly consist of a central line although trans-oesophageal Doppler is becoming more commonplace. While a central line provides useful information during the operation, using it post-operatively will also help to guide fluid management for a number of days post-op. With the advent of surgically run HDUs, your involvement with these monitors is increasing and you need to ensure you understand how to use them to best effect. They will be covered in more detail in STEP™ Foundation Module 3.

Patient monitoring

In this section we shall look at the range of things that the anaesthetist can and often does monitor. You will find out which parameters are of most importance for monitoring the cardiorespiratory systems and which other physiological parameters are of value to the anaesthetist in the perioperative period. The importance of this to you is that you are now required to look after extremely sick patients either on the ward or in an HDU. These patients will require all this monitoring and you must understand what you are using to be able to use it most effectively.

Look, listen and touch are watchwords for the anaesthetist and although a finger on the pulse may seem rather simple in today's technological world, it can still give the anaesthetist a vast amount of information. The array of electronic devices does not replace observing the movement of the chest wall, listening to the breath sounds using a stethoscope or looking at the fingers for adequacy of perfusion and cyanosis.

This principle holds true for the evaluation of sick patients on the ward. We are tempted to get lots of fancy equipment and tests, but so much can be gained from simple examination and touching the patient, for example pulse, temperature, perfusion, capillary refill, colour and urine output.

While there is an agreed minimal level of monitoring which all patients receiving general anaesthesia should have (and this level of monitoring is increasing from year to year), the nature of the surgery or the patient's general health may determine that more sophisticated monitoring be used.

We shall start by looking at this basic minimal monitoring and move onto more sophisticated methods in the next section.

Learning exercise	122

A fit 38-year-old man is due to undergo a laparoscopic cholecystectomy. What basic monitoring will the anaesthetist use to assess his cardiovascular system?

Learning exercise	123

For the same man what will be used to assess the respiratory system and the adequacy of ventilation?

Learning exercise	124

Apart from heart rate and blood pressure what simple measure would give information about the adequacy of organ perfusion (not necessarily in the case of a laparoscopic cholecystectomy)?

Learning exercise	125

Blood is not the only thing which the patient may 'lose' during prolonged surgery. Burns patients, children (especially neonates), and those having thoracotomies are particularly vulnerable to heat loss. Why is this important and how may it be prevented?

See answers to learning exercises on page 198.

Now try clinical case 17, which covers a major case throughout an operation.

 Clinical case 17

Mr E. Davies is a retired Welsh schoolteacher, aged 72 years, who has a 6.3 cm infrarenal abdominal aortic aneurysm which requires surgery. He is an insulin-dependent diabetic and takes nifedipine and thiazide diuretic to control his blood pressure. He gives the history of a 'small heart attack' three years ago but denies any angina, and has no orthopnoea or nocturnal dyspnoea.

On examination his chest is clear, his BP is 165/90 mmHg and his preoperative ECG shows signs of an old inferior myocardial infarct. His urea and electrolytes show a degree of renal impairment with the creatinine at 140 mol/l and urea of 13.6 mol/l. His blood count is normal with an Hb of 12.3 g/dl, and his blood glucose is slightly elevated at 11.2 mol/l.

Q1 What aspects of his history are particularly relevant?

You are seeing him on his arrival on the ward two days prior to surgery.

Q2 What are your main preoperative management goals for this patient?

The anaesthetist has seen the patient and prescribed temazepam as a premed. In addition he has crossed off the heparin you have prescribed.

Q3 What are his reasons for these actions?

The patient is now asleep and will obviously be monitored thoroughly.

Q4 Look at the following modes of monitoring. Decide which you feel is mandatory for this case and which is optional:
- ECG;
- non-invasive BP;
- arterial line—invasive BP;
- CVP line;
- Swan–Ganz catheter;
- urine output;
- pulse oximetry;
- temperature probe;
- capnography;
- blood glucose stick test.

Clinical case 17 answers

Q1 There is much to sort out here:
- Risk of coronary disease is high—vascular patient, old MI, diabetic, hypertensive.
- Major surgery is proposed thus increasing risk of complications.
- He has a mild degree of renal failure.

Q2 This is a high-risk procedure in a man with significant coexisting disease. You need to be thorough in your preparation. Particular note needs to be made of:
- starting a sliding scale preoperatively;
- informing the anaesthetists early to allow organization of ITU, consultant input, etc.;
- continue medication preoperatively—don't stop antihypertensive drugs;

Q3 The anaesthetist has prescribed a sedative premed to reduce the sympathetic drive preoperatively. Anxiety resulting in tachycardia and hypertension is undesirable in this patient.

It is common today to insert an epidural for perioperative and post-operative pain relief. If the patient has recently had heparin then there is an increased risk of epidural haematoma and an epidural is then contraindicated.

Q4

Table 19: Technique monitoring for Mr E. Davies

	Mandatory	Optional
ECG	☑	
Non-invasive BP	☑	
Arterial line invasive BP	☑	
CVP line	☑	
Swan–Ganz catheter		☑
Urine output	☑	
Pulse oximetry	☑	
Temperature probe	☑	
Capnography	☑	
blood glucose stick test	☑	

Answers to learning exercises

Process of general anaesthesia

115   Propofol has a very clear-headed and rapid recovery compared to thiopental (thiopentone) and is widely used in day-case anaesthesia as a consequence. It does not accumulate so much on repeat dosage and is often used as a continuous infusion. However, it is expensive and causes profound drops in blood pressure—not to be used on hypovolaemic patients.

Etomidate is less depressant to the myocardium and is ideally used in patients who are cardiovascularly unstable as it does not drop the BP as much as others. However, it is associated with significant adrenal suppression. Thiopental (thiopentone) is the oldest and best understood agent—and it is cheap. It can drop the BP considerably, may induce anaphylaxis and bronchospasm, and leaves quite a hangover.

116   The cardiovascular and respiratory systems are both depressed to varying degrees by the two most frequently used drugs. The resultant effects are hypotension due to both myocardial depression and peripheral vasodilation, and apnoea secondary to depression of the respiratory centre in the brainstem.

117   These effects, in particular the hypotension, are far more pronounced when the patient is hypovolaemic or has a significant reduction in cardiac reserve. This may frequently occur with emergency surgery and is why anaesthetists are always so obsessive about volume resuscitation prior to surgery. It may be irritating to the surgeon to have to wait, but without it the patient could easily arrest once anaesthetized. Patients with obstruction of the GI tract or those with GI bleeding are often hypovolaemic and in particular have intravascular volume depletion. Profound falls in BP may therefore occur at induction of anaesthesia. Adequate resuscitation is therefore essential.

118   Anaesthetic agents vasodilate patients and cause a drop in the BP. If the patient is hypovolaemic and maintaining their BP by vasoconstriction, the induction of general anaesthesia without rehydration will cause a catastrophic drop in BP and possibly

▼

arrest. That extra half an hour may prove a life saver.

119 The most basic would be a simple face mask ± airway. We have now moved on to the LMA which frees up the anaesthetist's hands but is essentially the same as a simple face mask but just pushed a bit further down. The third method would be intubation.

120 It is particularly important for many procedures today to have muscle relaxation. In days gone by this was provided by administering large amounts of general anaesthetic agent, which culminated in severe and profound side effects leading to death! Even though our modern general anaesthetic agents are safer to use, we still avoid using excessive amounts by ensuring that the muscle relaxation is provided by muscle relaxants and the anaesthetic agents are used only to keep the patient asleep.

121 Intubating the patient secures the airway and prevents any stomach contents entering the lungs, and allows us to ventilate the lungs without a leak when muscle relaxation has been used. The LMA is enormously useful as an airway device but it does not protect the airway. It is not a substitute for intubating the patient.

Patient monitoring

122 Basic monitoring should include:

- **Heart rate**—this can be measured peripherally (from the non-invasive blood pressure recorder such as a Dinamap or by the pulse oximeter) or centrally from the ECG; in certain cardiac conditions such as fibrillation there may be different readings from the two techniques.
- **Pulse oximetry**—this is usually considered a monitor of respiratory function but if peripheral perfusion is poor it does not function correctly, so it is indirectly a monitor of the CVS.
- **NIBP** will be measured intermittently using the Dinamap. For an operation such as this there is no need for any more invasive measure of BP.
- **ECG**—ECG is certainly a basic requirement as it gives information on heart rhythm and myocardial ischaemia as well as heart rate, depending on how the leads are configured. CVP, Swan-Ganz recordings and cardiac output measurement are more advanced and would not be used for this case.

123 **Capnography:** The physiological variable which measures adequate ventilation most closely is the arterial tension of carbon dioxide (p_aCO_2). This is because the p_aCO_2 is inversely related to the level of ventilation (the greater the ventilation the more CO_2 is cleared and so the lower the p_aCO_2). However, it is not routine anaesthetic practice to measure arterial blood gases as this is invasive, requiring arterial puncture. We therefore rely on capnography or measurement of the end tidal CO_2 level in the exhaled gas from the patient's lungs, which we use as an approximation of the p_aCO_2.

Pulse oximetry is a poor and late indicator of ventilation. Oxygen can still be passed from the alveoli to the blood with only minimal respiratory effort.

Oxygenation is therefore fine but ventilation is not. One of the tests of brainstem death is apnoeic oxygenation when no ventilation takes place but oxygen still diffuses across the lung.

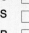

C ☐
S ☐
R ☐

124 Urine production in the kidney is very dependent on adequate renal perfusion therefore hourly urine output measurement is useful in this respect. Perfusion or blood flow to the major organs of the body, namely the brain, heart, kidneys and liver, is of paramount importance during any form of surgery but particularly during procedures where blood loss may be large or during prolonged surgery.

125 Heat loss is important as post-operatively this results in shivering which increases the oxygen demand of the body and necessitates supplementary oxygen therapy. After major surgery hypothermia may also affect cardiovascular stability and blood clotting. It can be ameliorated by:

- warming intravenous fluids (and any other washout fluids used);
- warm ambient temperature in theatres or recovery room;
- humidification of inspired gases.

Summary

The preparation of patients for planned procedures is evolving rapidly and there are many drivers for change in this complex area. Traditionally patients were admitted to hospital well in advance of their procedure, fully clerked by a member of the medical team, the appropriate investigations arranged and carried out and also assessed by the anaesthetist and surgeon scheduled to be involved in their procedure. Now patients are admitted on the day of the operation and are likely only to be seen by their anaesthetist and surgeon shortly before the procedure. It is therefore essential for patient safety that these individuals are properly prepared for their procedures as far in advance as possible.

Many hospitals are developing multidisciplinary Pre Operative Assessment (POA) Clinics. Patients are seen in these clinics by pre-assessment nurses, doctors, pharmacists, physiotherapists and other specialists as soon as possible after the decision that a procedure is necessary has been made. Each hospital you work in will have a slightly different system for the preparation of patients for planned procedures and therefore your role in this important area is also likely to vary. This Unit has discussed the importance and impact of co-existing disease in these patients and how particular conditions may affect the perioperative course. You should now be able to clinically assess patients appropriately, organise investigations, identify those at increased risk and refer them as necessary for specialist advice and also ensure that antibiotic and thromboprophylaxis guidelines are followed. If you have the opportunity to work in a multidisciplinary POA clinic you will find that you can all learn from each other and that an efficient pre-assessment process helps to alleviate some of the unpleasantness for patients who are required to undergo a diagnostic or surgical procedure.

Index